Advanced Tai Chi Chuan for Real Self-Defense!

Kung Fu forms, applications and fighting drills!

Al Case

Make sure you get the first book in this series,

*with **five hours** of video training:*

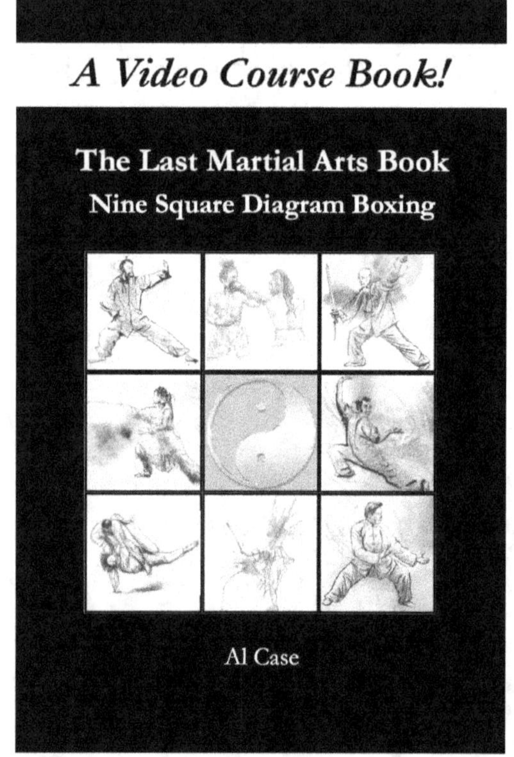

Table of Contents

Introduction

This is a book of very condensed Tai Chi Chuan.

Moves which are stylistic and don't have much application have been taken out. Only the combat applicable moves are left.

The moves are arranged on a nine square diagram, allowing for intense repetition. Repetition to the point of meditation.

This creates a very modular approach for learning, much like Pa Kua Chang, and makes learning incredibly fast and easy.

The techniques are based on the basic ten arm positions in the martial arts, and can be put together in a variety of effective techniques.

Everything relates to the combat training methods.

This makes it the easiest, most useful and combat workable method of Tai Chi Chuan in existence.

This book is also the second book on Nine Square Diagram Boxing.

While you can certainly study this book alone, I would advise getting my first book: The Last Martial Arts Book: Nine Square Diagram Boxing.

This book contains the only form in that art, all the applications, and the specific methods of training one how to use Tai Chi Chuan in combat.

This book presents the only form in the art of Nine Square Diagram Boxing.

Al Case

section one

Summation of Basics

In the martial arts there are no 'secret' or 'advanced' techniques.

There are only better basics.

Chapter One

Overview of Art

My arts follow a certain logic, but they do overlap, and you deserve a short word on how my art is arranged.

Matrixing is a scientific method which makes karate logical and easy to learn and easy to apply.

The mind likes what is simple. That is why traditional arts take decades to learn, and mine takes a couple of months.

Once one has learn how to matrix, they should apply those principles to every other art, this brings all arts together.

I have demonstrated how to apply matrixing to other arts through a variety of books and courses.

I spent a lot of time dissecting such arts as Tai Chi Chuan, the eventual result being 'Nine Square Diagram Boxing.' This is the second book about Nine Square Diagram Boxing, I recommend you get the first one, The Last Martial Arts Book: Nine Square Diagram Boxing.

Nine Square Boxing eliminates mysticism and makes Tai Chi Chuan simple and easy to work.

The book you are holding has the only form in Nine Square Diagram Boxing. As implied, it is Tai Chi, but based on combat effective postures, and not on the 'health building' or mystical aspects of that art.

After over 50 years in the arts it is one of the only forms I do religiously, and every day. The other is a form of Sanchin, but a Sanchin modified to explore the Slap Grab technique, and which includes Seisan in its moves.

The third art I have spent time constructing is 'Monkey Boxing.' This is a very intense course on how to go from weapons to fists to take downs. It is also incredibly simple as it is based on eight simple hand patterns.

The patterns are used, and expanded, from weapons to hands and take downs. They are interchangeable.

Thus, all of my arts are modular, the student can arrange the simple basics in a vast variety of techniques, all of which are useful in combat.

By simplifying the arts to functional basics I have sped up the time to enlightenment.

In this day of violence and societal unrest enlightenment is often overlooked, but it is probably the most important thing I can offer you.

Chapter Two

Warm Ups

In Matrixing the theory of warm ups is very simple. There are three directions, X, Y and Z. Using this for a base, applying it to the human body, one only needs to do a small number of stretches to achieve a degree of stretch in the three directions.

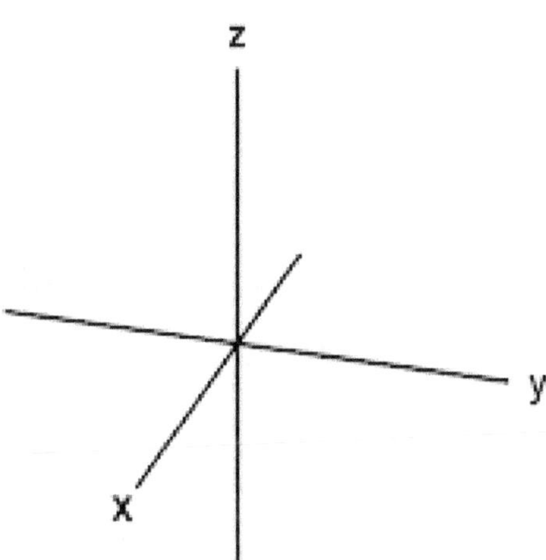

The stretches don't adhere exactly to the three directions, as the human body doesn't adhere to the three directions. I do the following exercises before every work out.

The first is the toe touch.

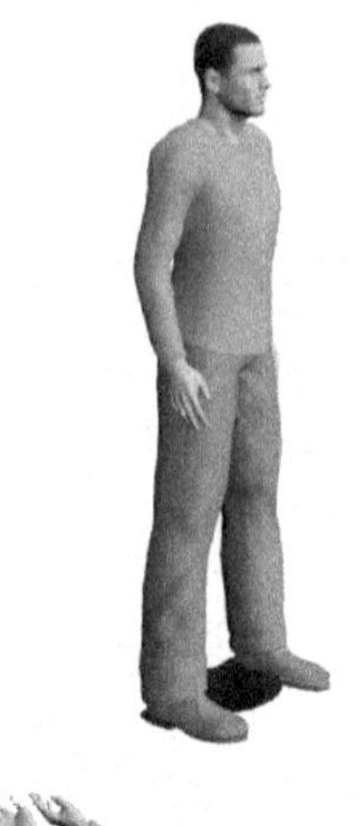

From a standing position lean back as if reaching for something behind you.

Bend at the waist and touch your toes, or the ground, or, as you get better, place your palms flat upon the ground, etc.

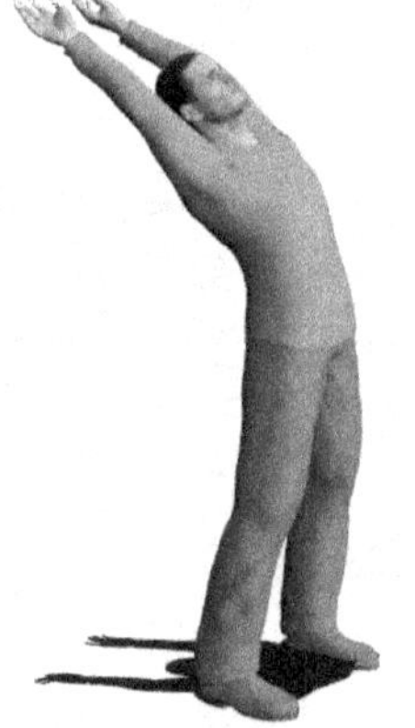

Don't bounce, don't strain, just hang. If you need more bend don't do it with physical effort. Do it by relaxing, letting the arms and body hang over the edge of your hips, and imagine a point deep in the earth.

This stretches the spine forward and back.

Ten reps is sufficient.

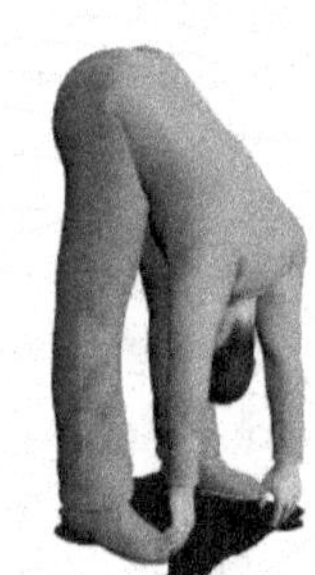

The second is the twist.

From a standing position twist the body to one side.

Turn to the other side.

This turns the spine right and left. Do not force or bounce.

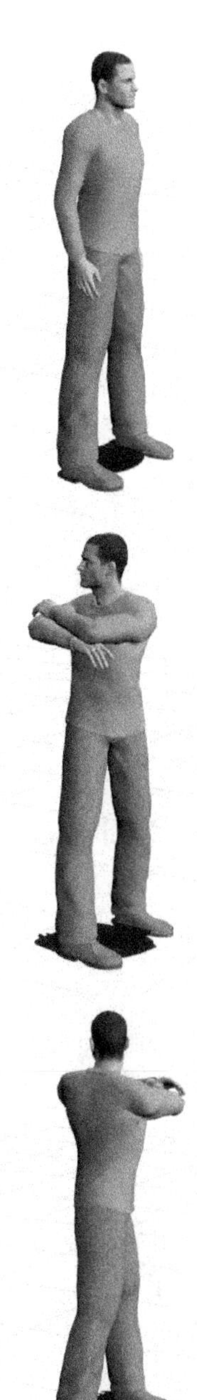

This is excellent for keeping the disks in place, and you'll notice the rest of the body is being tuned up. The arm joints, the knee joints, the ankles and the wrists, everything is bending slightly, but without undue effort, or without the exertion that might cause damage.

The idea her is not to do strength exercises for a body merely warming up. The idea is simply to wake up the joints to be used in a very light manner.

Ten reps is sufficient.

The third is the squat.

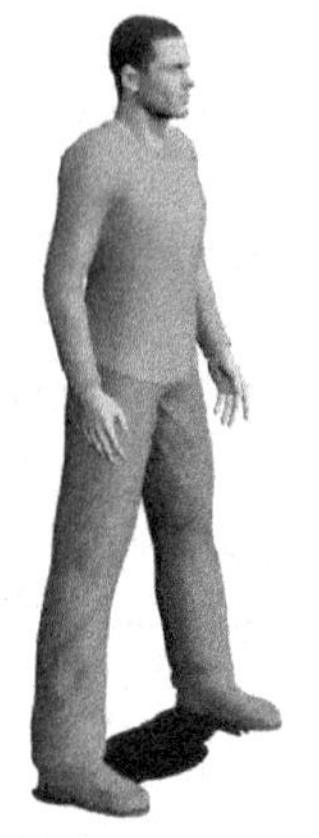

From a standing position bend at
the knees and touch the fingers to
the ground.

My software program won't show
the complete bend, but the fingers
touch the ground.

You can spread the feet for this
one, even as wide as a horse
stance.

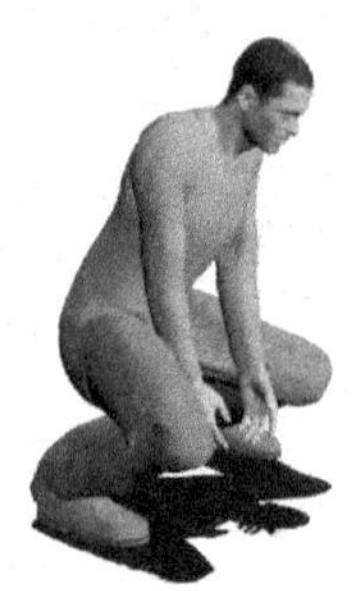

You will want to explore the
'pointing outwards' of the feet
until you find your ideal foot
position.

Half the body's height is in the legs.
Thus, the legs need a little extra. This is first a strength exercise, but also an
aerobic exercise.

While ten reps is sufficient, I used to do 500 of these a day. Just make sure
you work up to it. Ten a day for a week. 20 a day for another week. 30 a day
for a week. Keeping adding ten each week until 50 weeks have passed.

After this drill I do leg raises front and side, push ups, or any other simple
exercises that build the body up and prepare it for the martial arts.

Chapter Three

The Form

The Form in Nine Square Diagram Kung Fu is very simple.

Breath to the tan tien (the one point), which is the body energy generator.

Sink the weight down the legs. Cause weight to make work to make energy.

Energy Formula

Weight = Work= Energy

Turn the hips into the action, or into alignment.

Have 'unbendable arms.' These are arms which are slightly bent, not tensed, but empty, and visualize energy flowing through them, in every technique.

You can shoot a straight arm, but you risk over extending yourself and giving the opponent a lever.

Chapter Four

Form, Technique, Chaos

The Theory of Techniques is that they are the bridge between the perfect idea of the form, and the chaos of the world.

One must achieve the correct body alignment in the techniques, thus enabling the power to run from the ground to the block, or punch, and into the target.

One must learn to synchronize (harmonize) all body motions so they start at the same time, so they end at the same time in the culmination of a strike.

This is the application of CBM, Coordinated Body Motion, to the motion of the body.

This includes breathing, sinking the weight, and so on.

Chapter Five

Freestyle

The Theory of Freestyle is not to fight, but to move at the same time, or before, and make your body a glove to the opponent's fist.

One must analyze one's body to understand the zones that might be attacked and how they are attacked.

One must analyze the opponent's body into weapons to be used and the solutions for the attacks.

One must become aware not of the hands, but of the shoulders, the hips, the tan tien.

Strikes emanate from the center of the body energetically, but before that, from the mind, and before that from the 'I am' of the individual.

One must focus one's eyes on the opponent's eyes, for the eyes are the windows to a man's soul.

Chapter Six

Nine Square Footwork

The footwork in the Nine Square is very simple. You simply walk a figure eight backwards on a diagram built of nine shoulder width squares. I'll show you that in the next couple of pages.

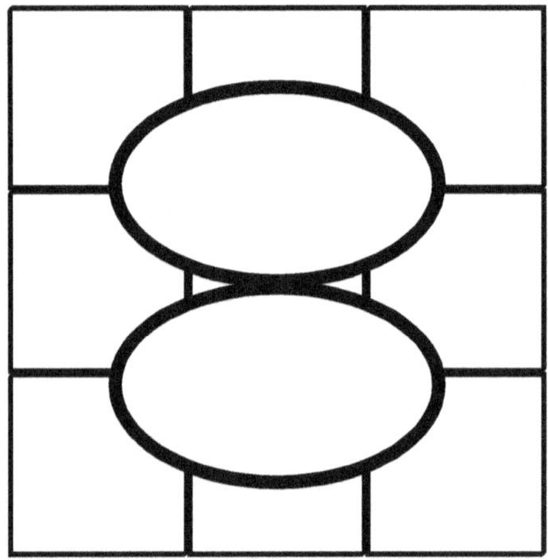

When stepping one should move slowly. For instance, feeling the weight go up the right leg, and down the left leg, up the left leg and down the right leg.

I used to imagine a tennis ball going up the tube of my leg to the tan tien, then down the other leg. Back and forth.

These days I simply feel the push from the leg doing the propelling.

It is VERY important to turn the hips into the action, or to align the hips with the body.

Chapter Seven

Form Footwork

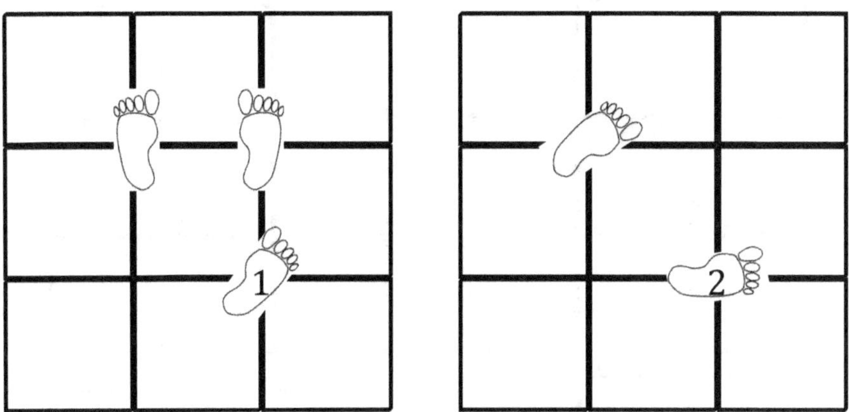

Simply follow the numbers in the feet in each diagram.

You will either step backwards, or pivot.

Remember, the important things are to go slowly and feel the weight going up and down your legs, feel the tan tien create energy, mentally guide the energy up to the arms.

The arms will make certain circular moves that tend to mimic the yin yang symbol.

I suggest learning the form, then doing the form with the eyes closed, trying to place the feet at the end of the form on the exact position from the beginning of the form.

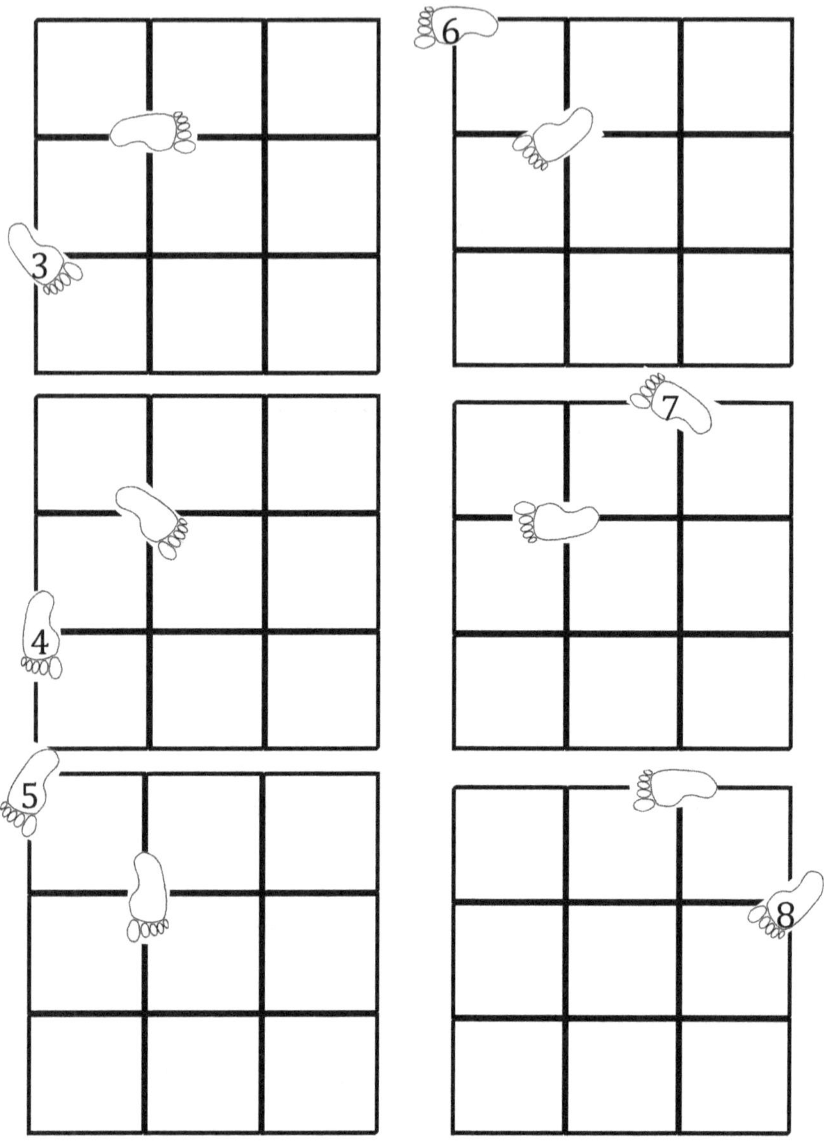

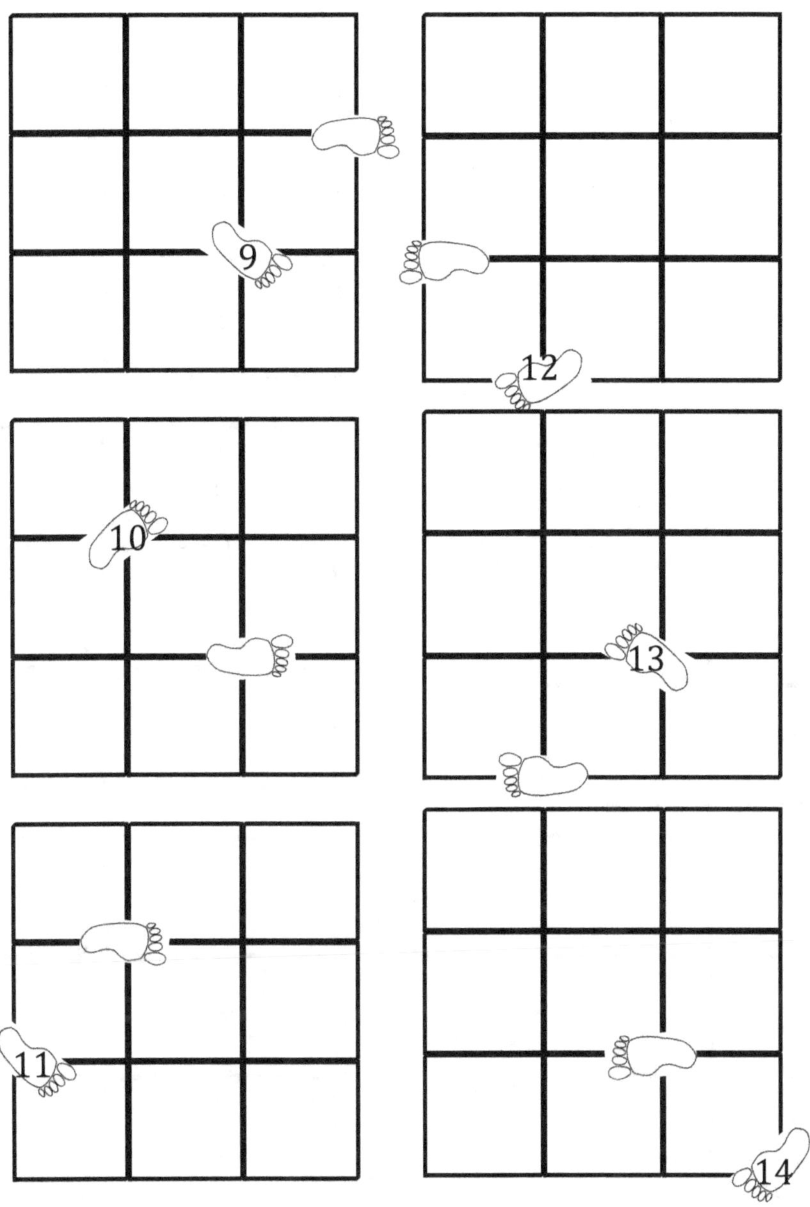
9
10
11
12
13
14

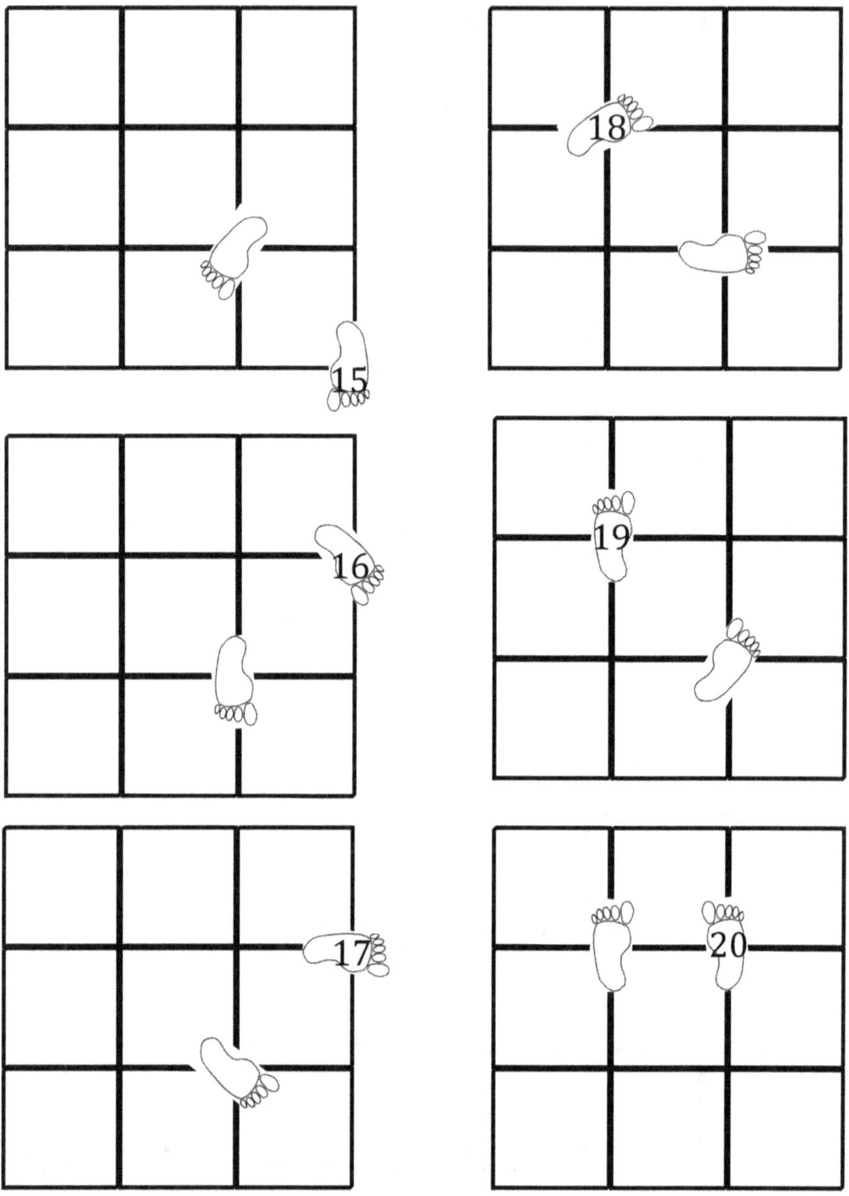

Chapter Eight

Circle of Blocks

The following Diagram, taken from an earlier book, represents the Circle of Blocks.

This shows how the various karate blocks are used in Karate, and other hard arts, to create a circle around, and protect, the body.

Nine Square Diagram Kung Fu is different, however. The defender moves back more, and the blocks tend to absorb more, rather than collide.

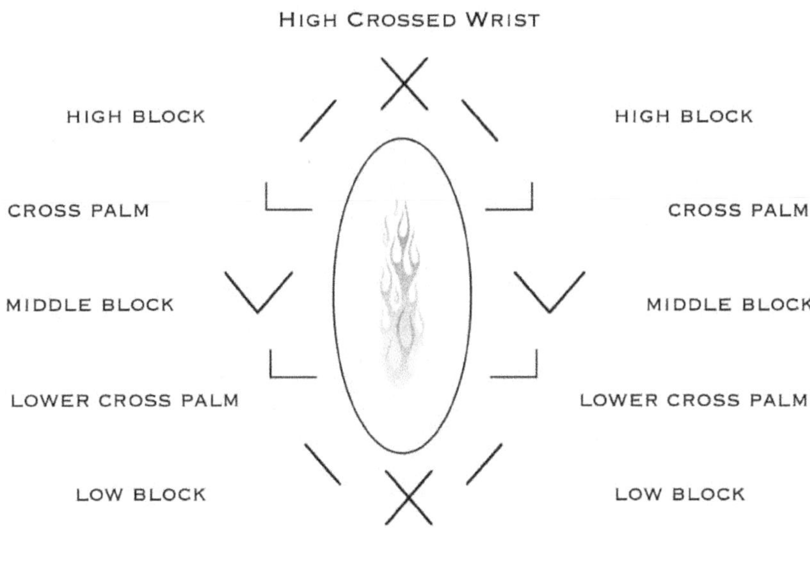

I always recommend a student learn a hard art like Matrix Karate first.

Chapter Nine

Angle of Attack

In Nine Square Diagram Kung Fu one visualizes oneself standing not just on a nine square footwork pattern, but with the nine square pattern imposed over the body.

One can better visualize areas to protect, and which areas can be protected by which weapons.

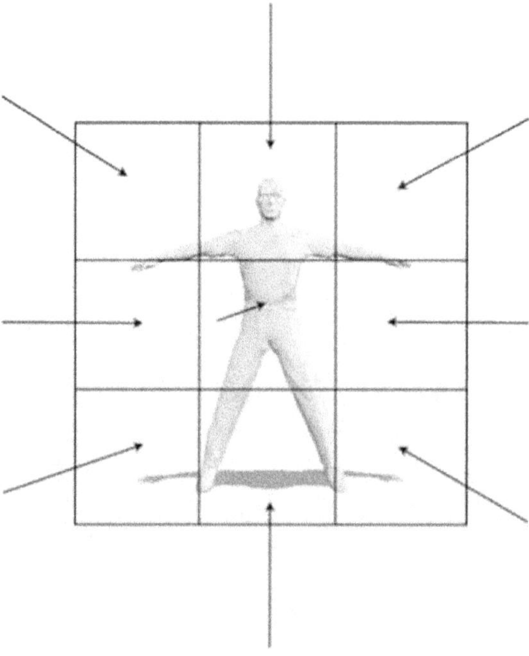

Chapter Ten

Ten Arm Positions

There are four basic blocks in karate. These positions can be translated into softer arts, such as Tai Chi or Nine Square, simply by visualizing the arm positions at angles to absorb, rather than to collide with the incoming force.

One can, of course, apply these ten arm positions whether you are moving in (attacking) or retreating (absorb and push)

You will find these ten arm positions in the form I am about to describe. They will be inside of larger moves, and they will look different than these karate manifestations.

But one should study a hard art before a soft art.

If one appreciates the reality of collision and pain first they will better understand the necessary movements to encircle, absorb, and otherwise manipulate the attacker.

I

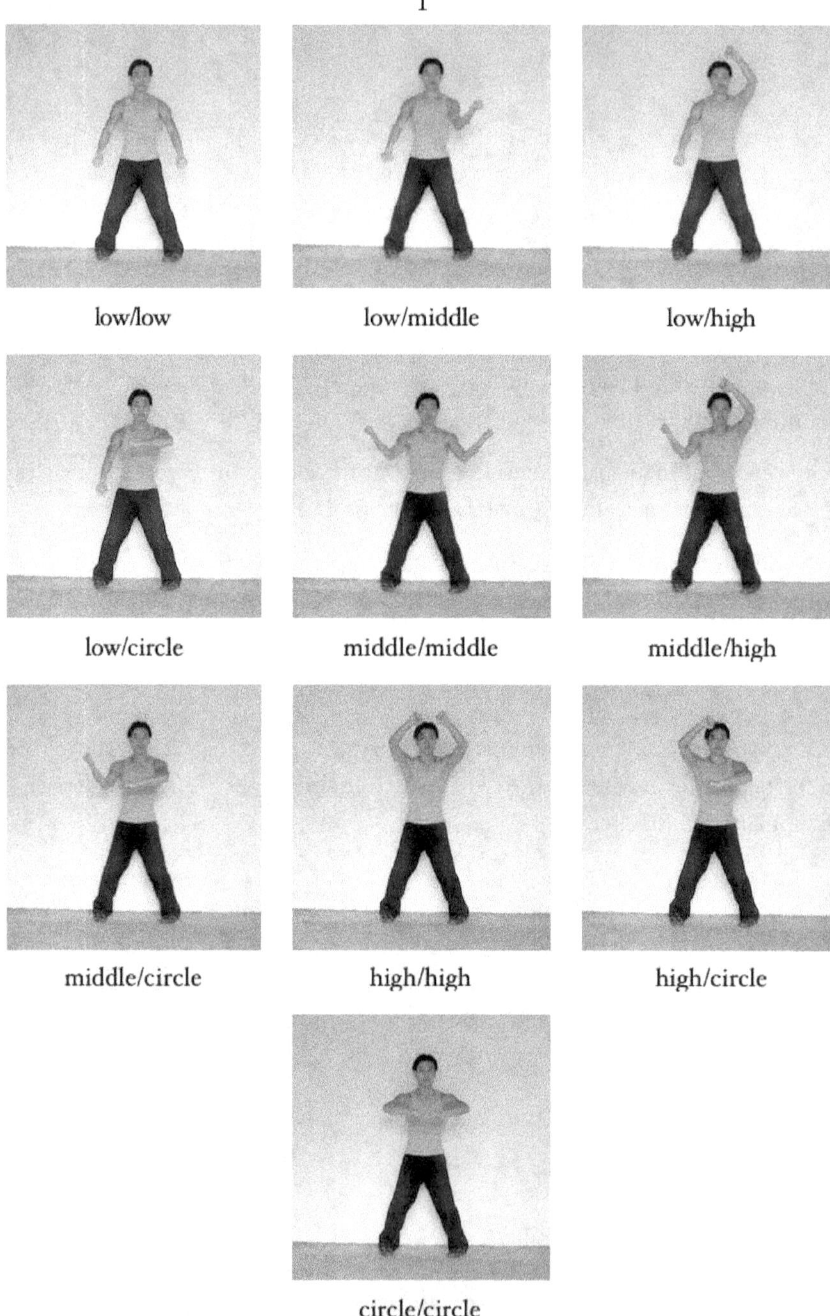

low/low   low/middle   low/high

low/circle   middle/middle   middle/high

middle/circle   high/high   high/circle

circle/circle

section two

The Form

I do the form with my eyes closed

to aid in the visualization of function.

Chapter Eleven

The Advanced Form

The form in this section is simple, but attention must be paid to the pushing of the legs, the turning of the hips into the action or into an alignment of the body, the circling of the arms so as to deal with the attack.

One must also pay attention to what per cent of the power comes from thrusting (the legs), turning (the hips/body alignment), and lowering the weight.

The following postures are known by a variety of names, and sometimes I have just substituted my own terms for them. The history of these postures is often interesting.

For instance, you don't really 'brush the knee,' the posture just resembles that motion.

And Fair Lady was originally Fair Lady Weaves at the Shuttles, and was a nifty, sort of complex motion of quick bird beak strikes, which sort of resembled a lady weaving at a shuttle.

In presenting these postures I have eliminated the fanciful and mythological and returned to a more functional positioning. No talk of mysterious chi, though that may well happen.

But if your chi manifests it will be because you understand the function and do practice your moves until the universe listens to you and does what you tell it to.

I recommend doing a hard art first, which is why I included the only hard form I do in the previous book, 'The Last Martial Arts Book.' It is called Sanchin, but I DO NOT do it the classical way. I do it a totally different way, I use a 'slap/grab' move that makes your techniques correct and functional.

When you do the form make sure you focus on when and why you thrust the legs or turn the hips or align the body.

Power comes from three things, thrust, rotate (turn) and dropping the weight (gravity). It helps to isolate what percentage of which power is in every single move.

But don't neglect to harmonize (CBM ~ Coordinated Body Motion) in not just the motions of the body parts, but in the application of the three powers. CBMing the three powers, thrust, rotation and gravity, will bring you to the fourth power: Intention.

The body can't manifest 'chi' unless the parts of the body are in coordination (harmony).

The following section, having to do with application/function, will help you understand that.

To do the form do the following moves in the order they are presented. Move slowly but with intention. Have the eyes closed and visualize energy and function.

Entering the Form

Raise and Lower

Stand square, raise the arms as you inhale for about five seconds.

Lower the arms as you exhale for about 10 seconds.

Four breaths a minute.

Raise the body slightly, an inch or two, with the raising of the arms.

Lower the body slightly, an inch or two, with the lowering of the arms.

Breath as if to the tan tien. Air goes to bottom of lungs, diaphragm lowers, energy wave goes down to the tan tien.

Tien tien creates energy.

If you stand relaxed, with the arms extended to the sides, you can feel your fingertips tingle with the cycle of energy through the body.

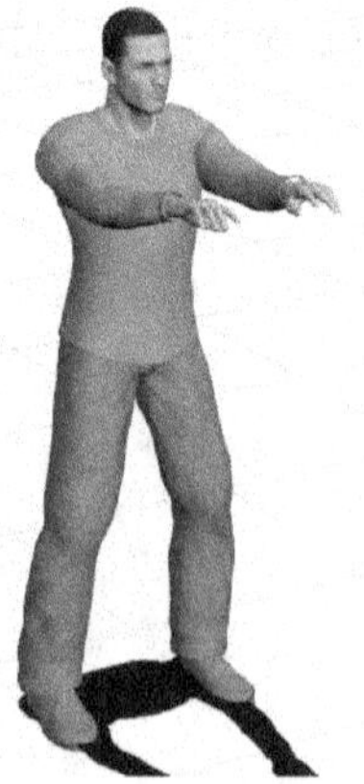 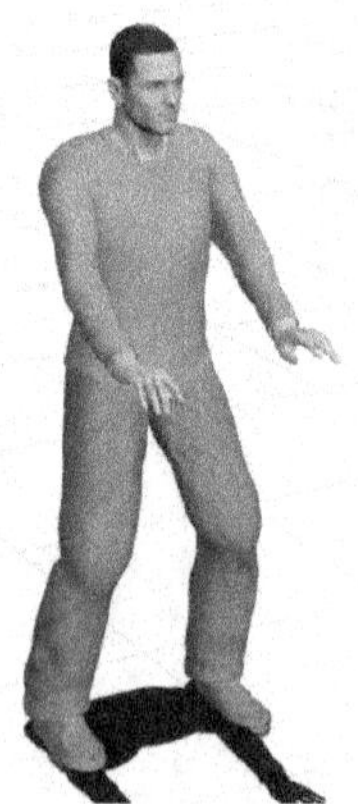

Entering the Form

Circle Slap

Stand with feet shoulder width apart, knees very slightly bent.

Circle one hand out as if slapping.

Circle the other hand out as if slapping, the first hand circles to be in front of the belly.

Have the legs bent slightly.

Turn the hips slightly.

Synchronize breathing.

Make the sweep of the hand, the turn of the hips as a singular, harmonious motion.

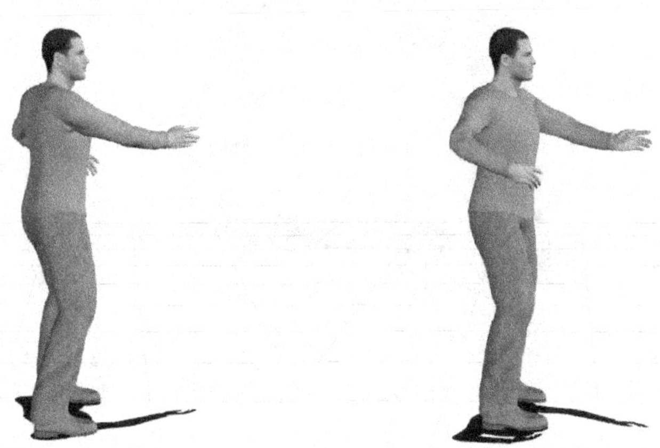

Move One

Roll Back

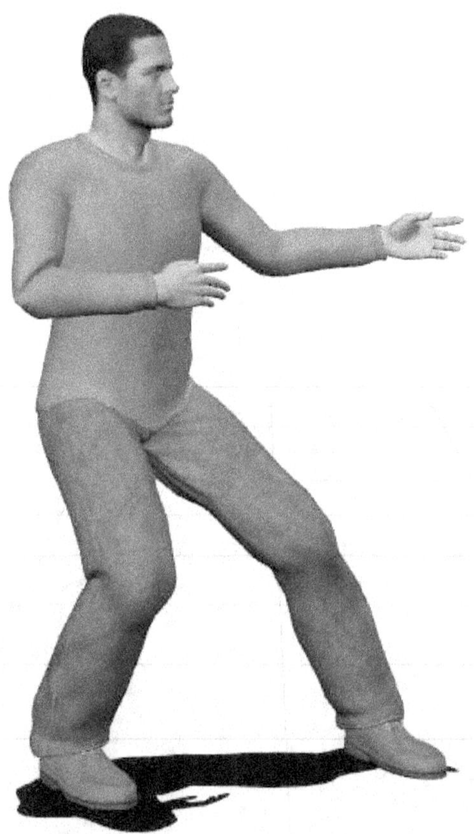

From the Circle Slap step back with the right foot and enter the Roll Back posture. Feet, hips and shoulders are in line. It's like pulling a rope.

Move Two

Brush Knee

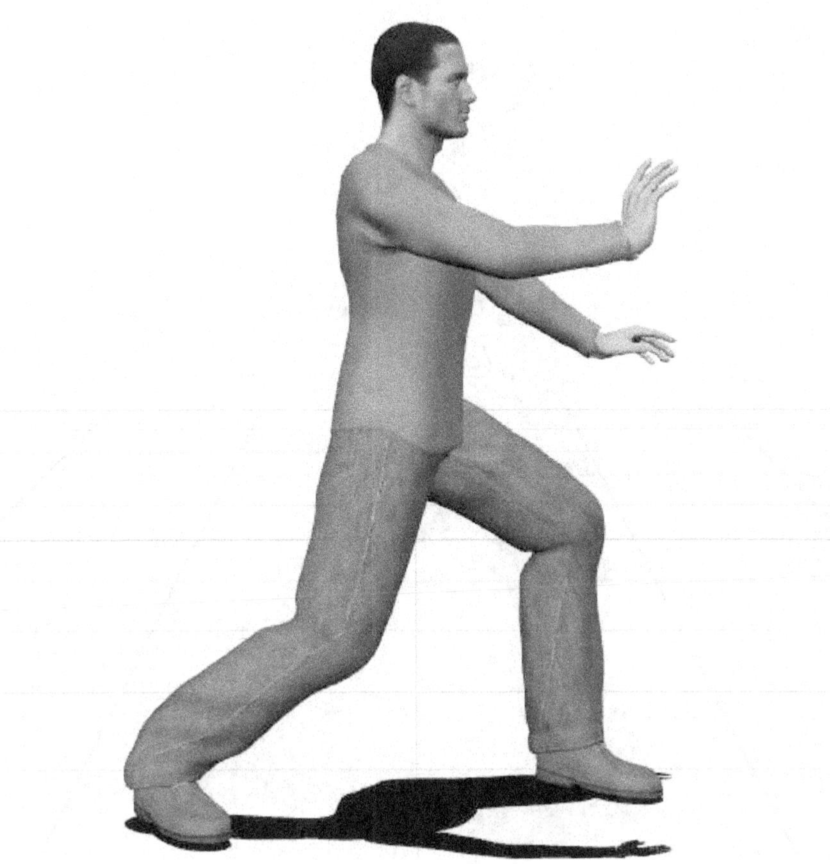

Bring the left hand over and down in a small circle as you execute a right palm push. Hips and shoulders turn into the strike. Push with the leg turn the hips, extend the arms like you're pushing a wall over.

Move Three

White Snake

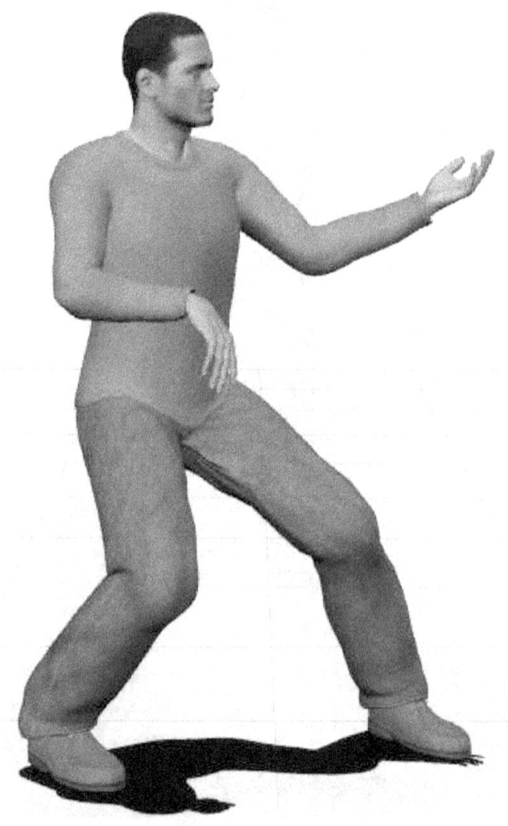

Shift into a back stance as you retract the right hand in a parry as you roll the left hand in and over to a left palm up block/spear. The motion of your hands will be mirrored by energy in your tan tien.

Move Four

Fair Lady

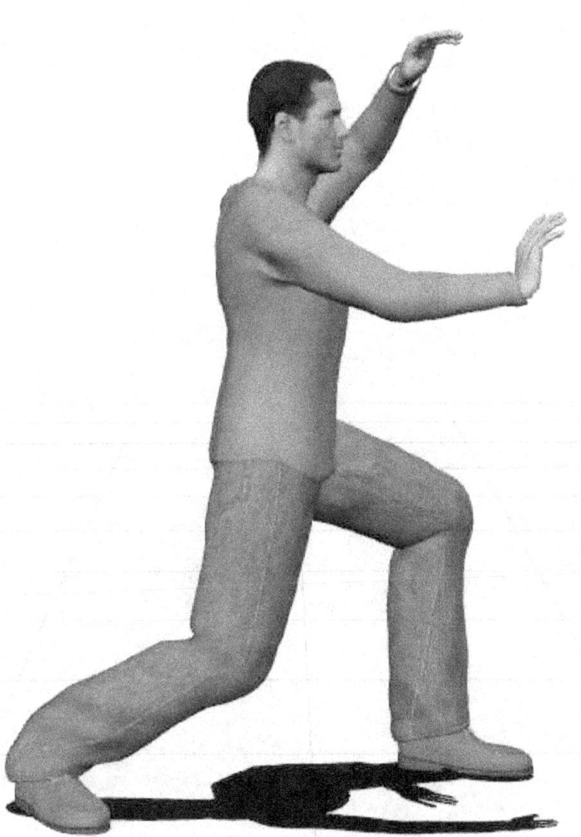

Shift into a front stance as you execute a left high block and a right palm thrust. Feel the energy go up and down your legs as you move.

Move Five

Inverted White Crane

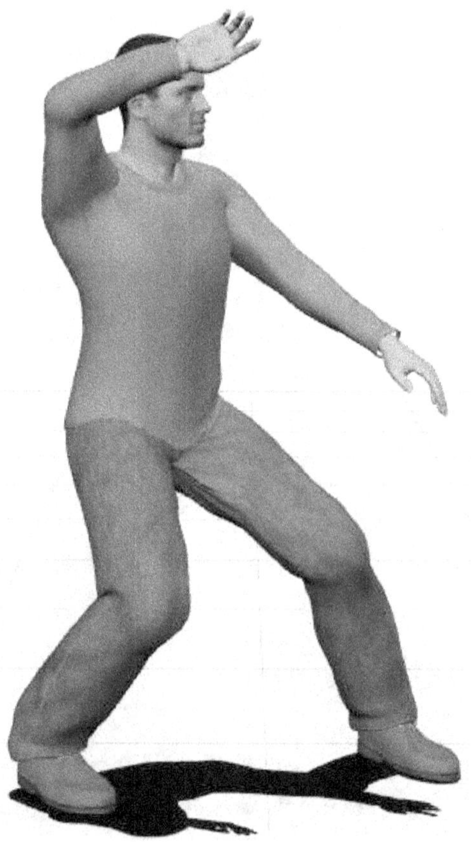

Shift into a back stance as you circle the left hand down in an inverted low block and the right hand up through a high block. The belly should always be taut. Not tight…but taut.

Move Six

Outblock

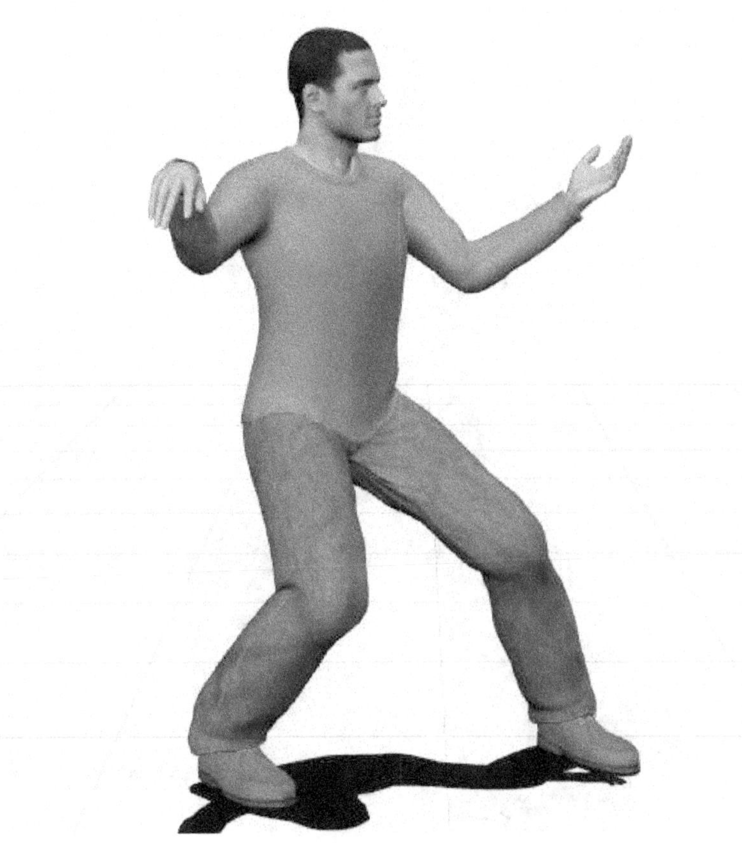

Sink the weight on the back leg and focus on alignment of the feet, hips, shoulders as you continue the circle of the right hand downward to a grab/ whip and execute a left outward block. Don't load up the tan tien with energy, feel the mix of yin and yang in concert with your hands.

Move Seven

Single Whip

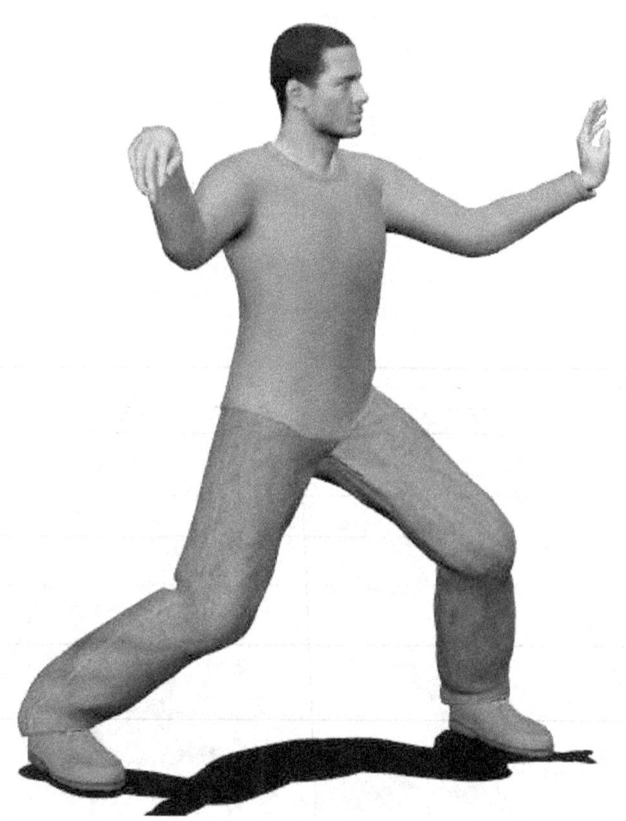

Keep feet, hips shoulders aligned as you shift forward and execute a left palm thrust. Do with closed eyes and it is easier to visualize an opponent.

Move Eight

Slap Low

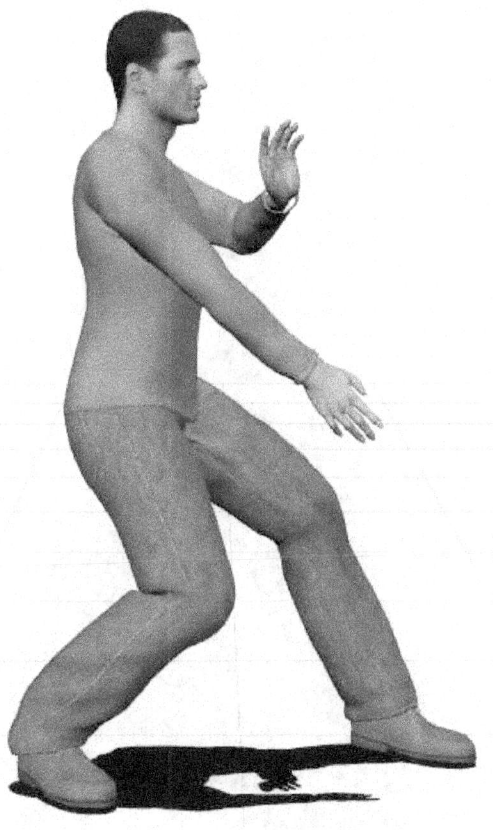

Shift back, turning the hips in as you slap low with the right hand and guard the face with the left hand Technically, this would be an 'Inverted Pole Position.' Do with closed eyes and it is easier to visualize your hands making shapes like sparklers in the dark.

Move Nine

White Crane

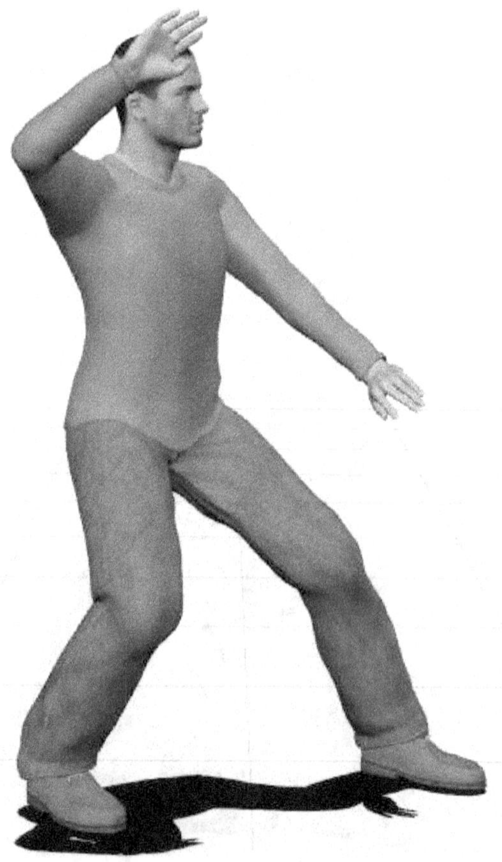

Pivot to the right on the back leg into a back stance as you continue the circling of the arms into a right high block and a left low block. Your hands should be endlessly curving, symbolizing the yin yang and interchanging the energy from side to side, from loop to loop.

Move Ten

Slap Low

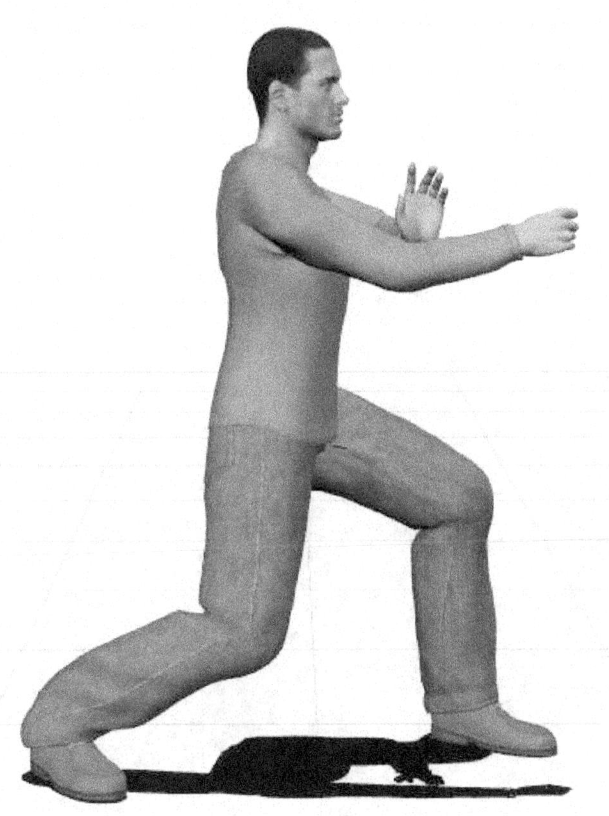

Continue the circling of the hands as you shift into a front stance. Execute a right punch and a left palm block. Retract with a bounce. Never leave a hand out to be grabbed and levered.

Move Eleven

Pole Position

Circle the right hand up and the left down (figure right) and keep circling to a left low slap and a right face guard. Synchronize your breathing, in and out, with the expansion and contraction of your body.

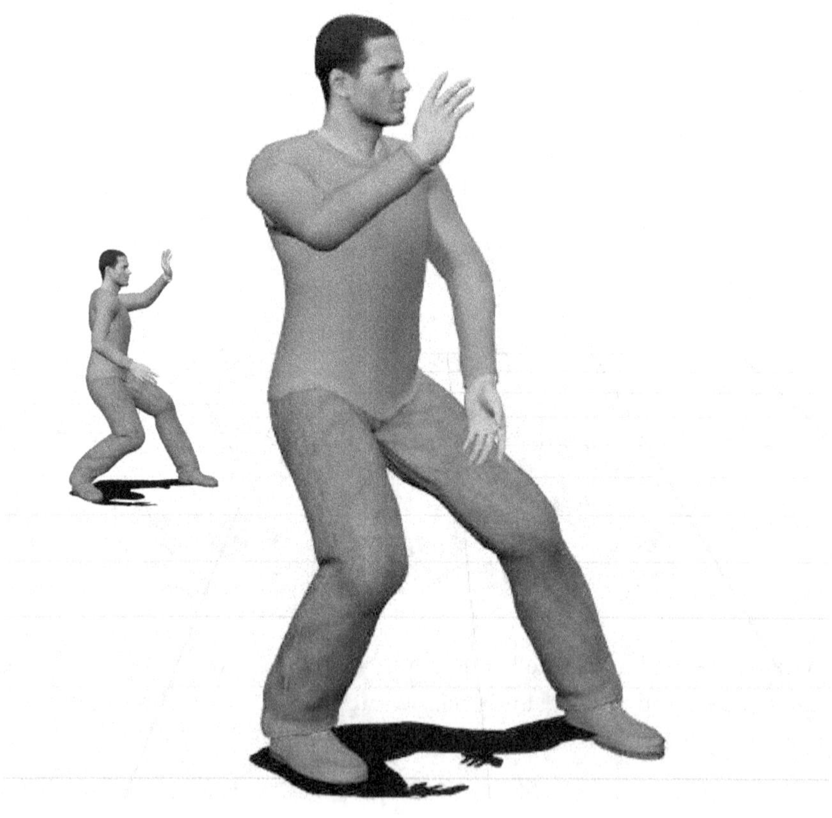

Move Twelve

Ward Off

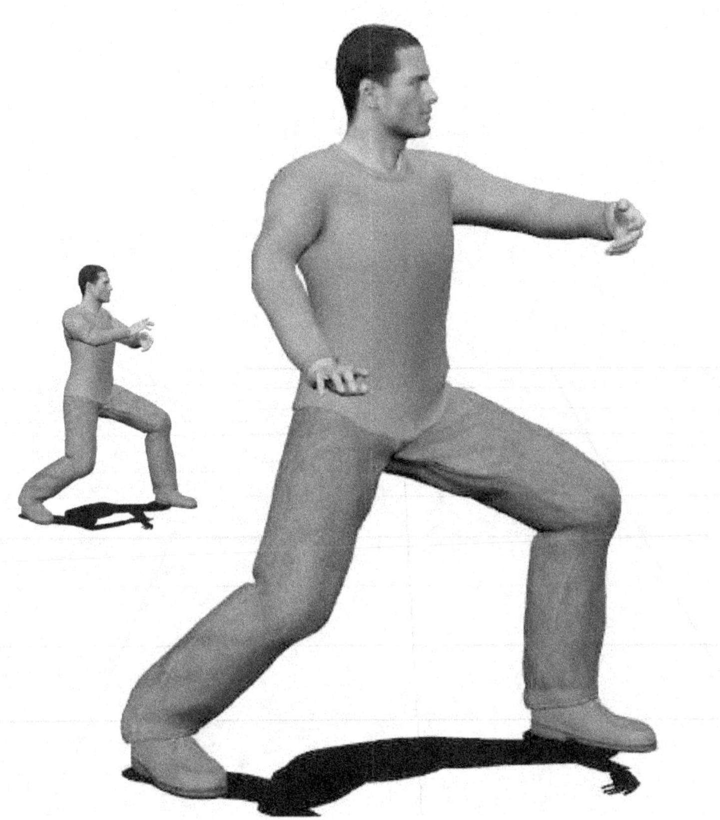

Shift to a front stance as you stroke across the wrist with the right hand (figure right) and open the left arm in a circle. Clear out the space around you.

44

Follow the Nine Square foot work pattern

by either pivoting or stepping back.

When you reach the end of the form

step up to the original position.

Chapter Twelve

Enlightenment

As I said, I do this form with my eyes closed.

I focus on footwork, making sure a pulse of energy, represented by weight, goes up and down the legs.

I focus turning the hips so they either go into the action, or set up the body alignment.

I concentrate on making the arms go in very yin yang like curves.

I become aware of the pulsing of energy as I do techniques.

I visualize attacks and handling them.

Most important…the most important thing I can tell you…is that you must do the form with your eyes closed.

Learn how to relax, even while pulsing and grounding. Synchronize the breath and…learn how to swim in space.

Remove thoughts of resistance, of gravity, and become apart from earthly matters. Feel the energy pulse through your legs and expand from the tan tien. Feel the energy in your arm positions.

This form normally take a while to feel the full effects

If you can free yourself from considerations, become separate from the universe and exist only in your own imagination, you will achieve a different and very much superior understanding of reality.

Your martial art will shine and forever work.

section three

Applications

The form is theory,

the techniques are application of theory,

freestyle is the application of theory in the middle of chaos.

Chapter Thirteen

The Techniques

Matrixing is a logical way of arranging martial arts knowledge, technique, and so on, in a way so that you have a large and usable database.

This enables one to simplify everything, and better access what moves you need when you need them.

However, as one progress into various arts they have to make choices. Do I go soft or hard, do I chose foot work over confrontation, and so on.

In the end one chooses those concepts and principles that best fit ones own person. This includes body, limitations, mentality, and so on.

And sometimes one must figure out how to blend certain arts, or when to use certain arts, or not use certain arts.

Nine Square Diagram is the result of my cogitations and explorations into this matter; it is the best solutions I could come up with to evolve the theory of form into the workability of the chaos of combat.

The basic principle here is that you will be either on the inside (of an attacker's arm) or the outside (of an attacker's arm), and that will guide your choices.

From those positions there are only so many things you can do, and it is those things that are at the heart of the Nine Square Diagram Kung Fu Techniques.

You must train, moving at the same time, until you develop your sixth sense.

Chapter Fourteen ~ Roll Back Pressure Points

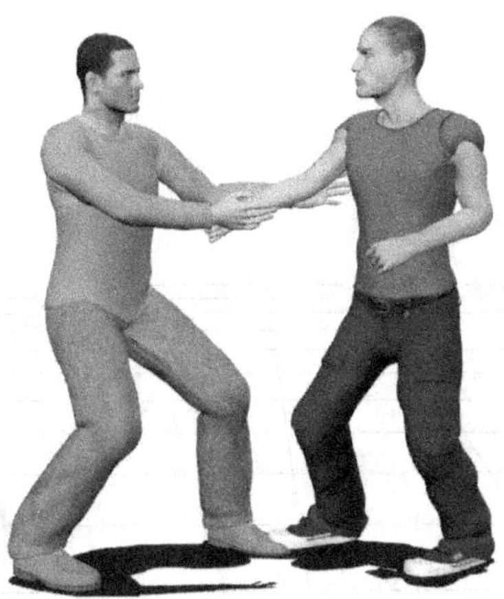

Step back and catch the attacker's arm with Roll Back.

This is a simple move wherein you move with the opponent, matching speed and guiding slightly.

Most punches will circle at the end, and if he does circle his punch he closes his body, giving you lots of targets while you have lots of weapons.

If he does punch straight, or even pushes, it can actually be easy to catch the arm like this.

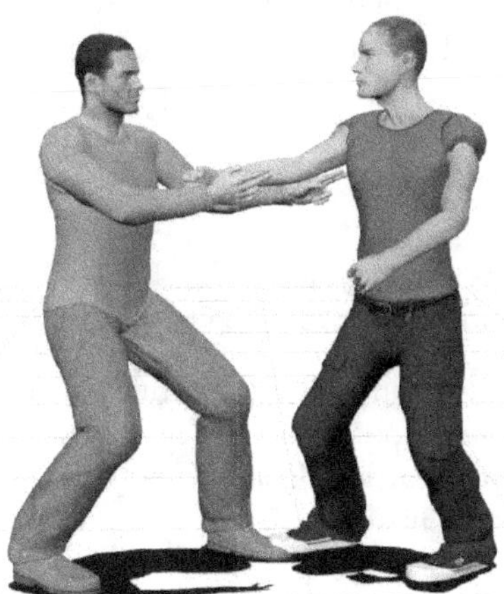

Lift his arm slightly and shoot your fingers into the axilla, the nerve cluster in his armpit. Make sure you strengthen your fingers greatly before shooting fingers. Your right hand can follow with a full body weight punch.

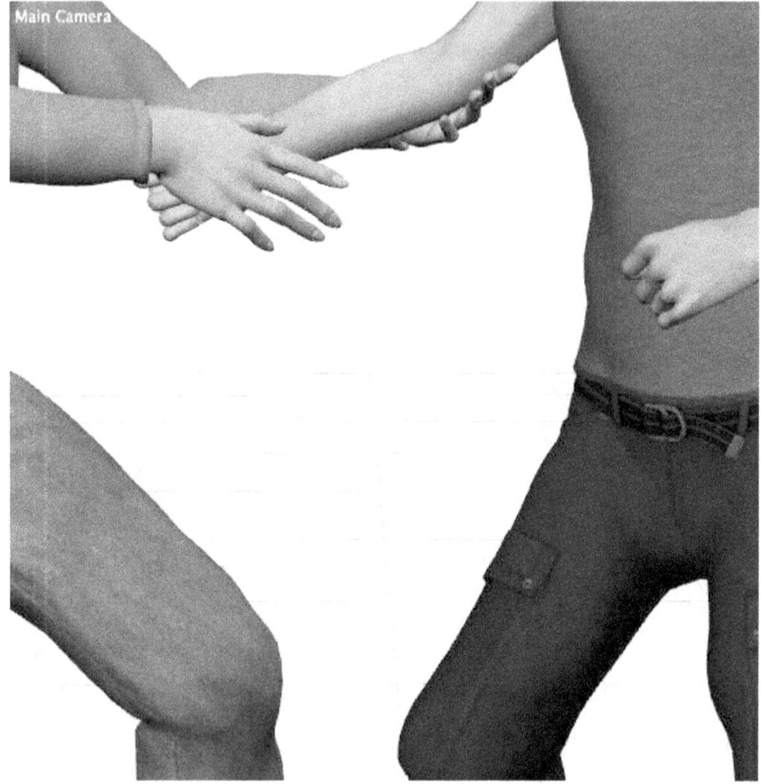

Also, you can turn his wrist slightly and press your thumb into the pressure point on the wrist, about two inches above the joint.

Pressure points are commonly found in indentations, called cavities. Don't attack the bulging 'armor' of a body, insert your fingers into the cavity and press.

You will find pressure points on the inside of the wrist, in the crotch of the elbow, on top of the radial nerve, and so on.

I don't spend a lot of time on pressure points. As you practice the art you will find them naturally, without effort. They are excellent for 'come alongs' when you don't want to joint lock somebody (risk damage to them? Some other reason?) and take them some place.

Roll Back and Uproot

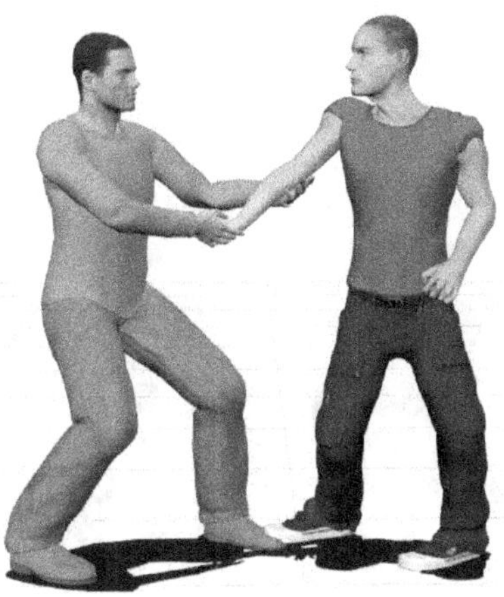

Another good method if to turn the opponent's arm palm up, lining up the wrist, elbow, shoulder and…the back shoulder!

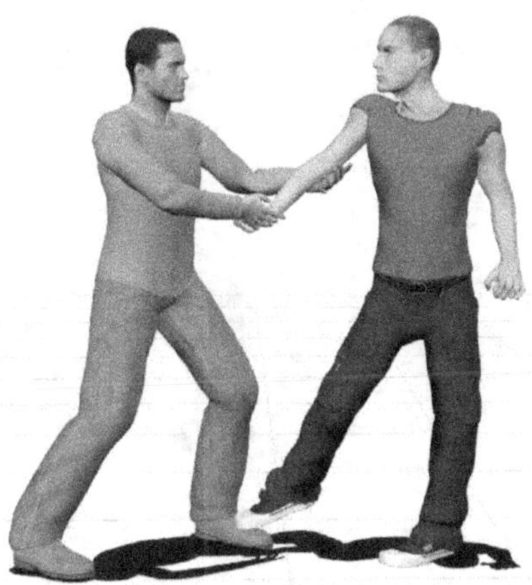

Push with your legs and whole body weight and push the arm up and back. If you keep his shoulders aligned he will fly away, an easy dozen feet. If he resists the push then pull him violently downward to the ground.

If his shoulders or elbow bend then you will have to contend with a body that is trying to wiggle out of the hold.

You will notice that you can combine attacks from these techniques, and even different techniques to make more techniques.

Roll Back and Break

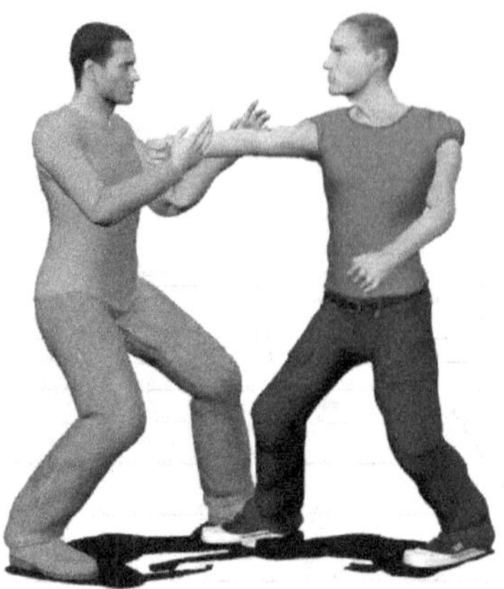

Use roll back to catch the attacker's arm.

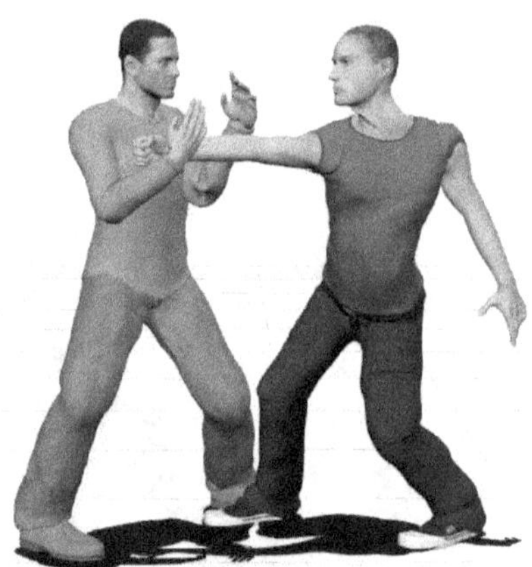

Turn into a horse stance, using hips power to break the elbow.

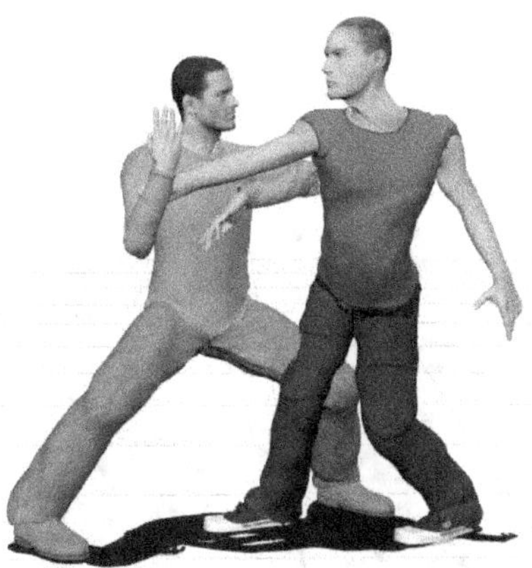

Shuffle into the opponent while controlling the arm and deliver an elbow spike to the axilla (the cluster of nerves in the armpit).

If you are taller then you can elbow the face.

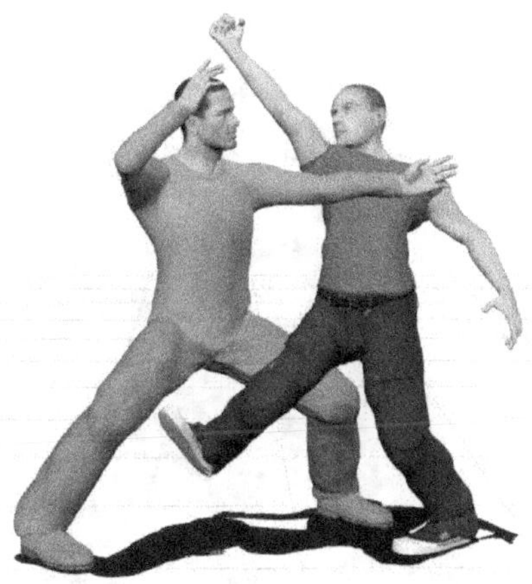

Extend the Left arm, sweeping his body back over your left leg. Watch out for his right hand. You don't want it smacking you in the face. Explore ways to lift it or move it so he can fall but can't grab a hold of you or flail into your face.

If you are taller you can sweep the arm across his face.

This is called a 'splitting' technique. The bottom goes one way, the top goes the other, and you 'split' the top half and the bottom half of the person.

Chapter Fifteen ~ Brush Knee and Push Shoulder

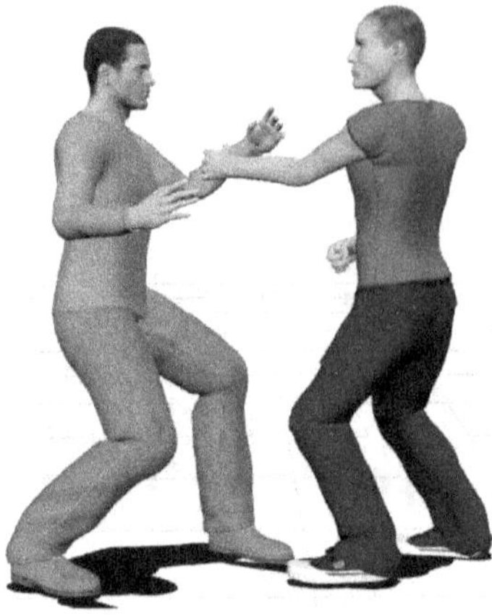

One of the. most functional Brush Knee Techniques takes into account the fact that the arm tends to circle at the end of a punch.

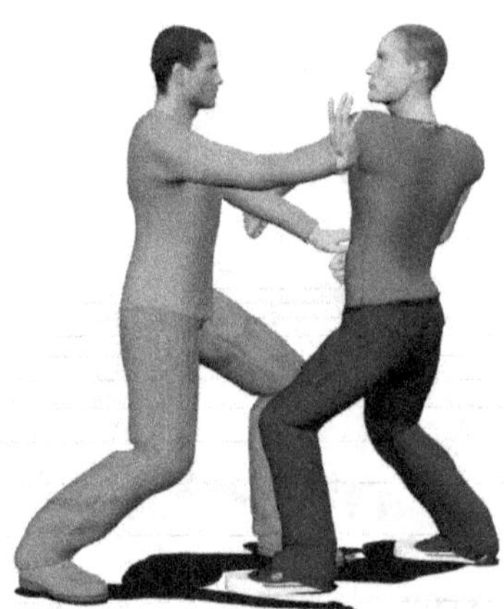

When you bring the hands up to catch the punch (roll back) go over the punch and let it pass as you bring the arm down in a parrying type of low block. Shuffle/shift forward and place the back hand on the shoulder and push upwards.

This unbalances the opponents and creates further openings.

One can also just use a fist and punch the face or the body.

Brush Knee and Palm Strike to Chest

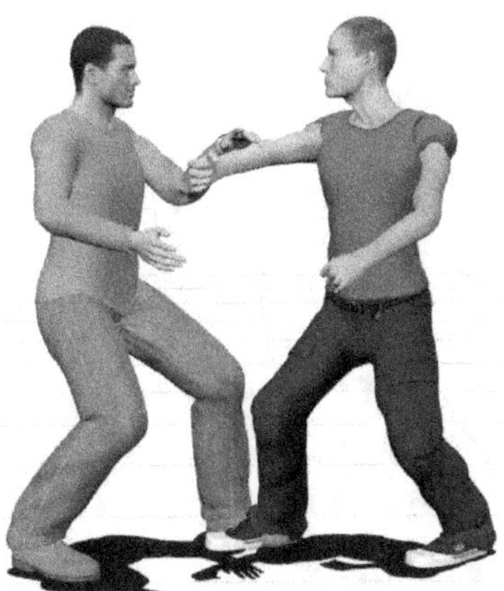

If you do Brush Knee on the other side you must guide the hand down and not let it circle at the end. This requires precision of harmony, as your arm must exactly match the speed and trajectory of your attacker's arm.

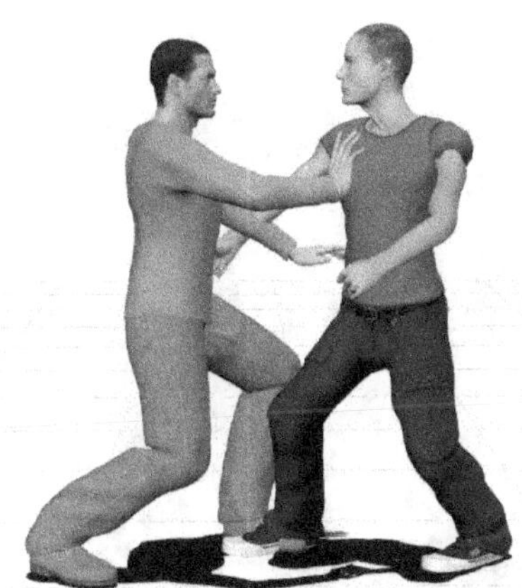

Parry/guide the attacker's arm down and to the side and shuffle forward. The palm strike to the chest must be done with a pulsing snap.

Be patient. there are many techniques here, so practice them until you can do them full speed with COMPLETE CONTROL!

The less of a danger you are to your partner, the more of a danger you will be to a real attacker.

Brush Knee and Oblique Kick

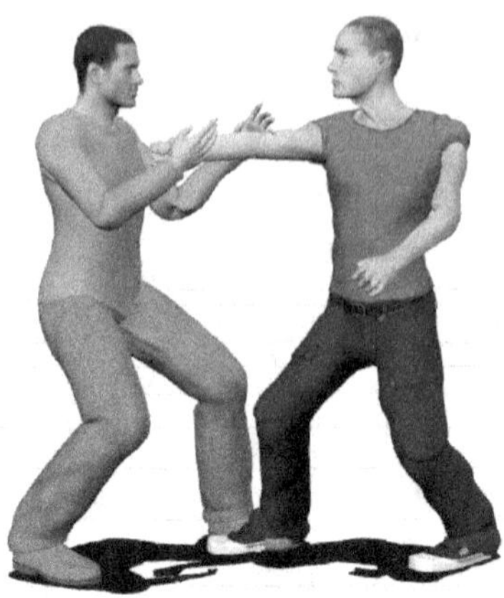

The last application for Brush Knee is to catch the arm and hold it. Do a quick change of the feet and stomp the attacker's forward knee. sideways. He should buckle nicely.

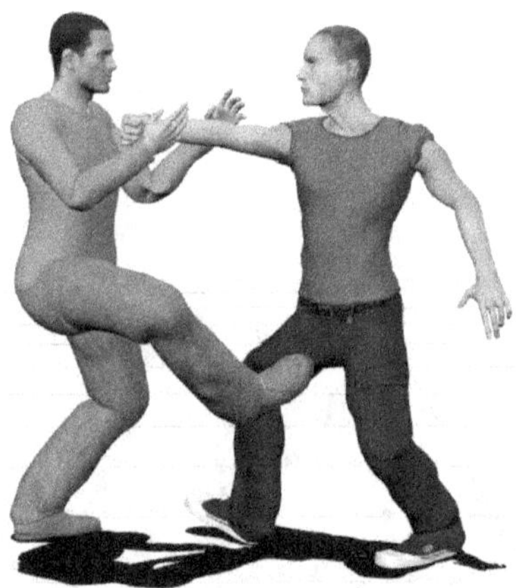

One could also kick the groin, kick the rear leg so as to dislocate the hip.

Obviously, there are many potentials here, so do not take the ones i have presented as the end all be all. Explore…and find more.

Chapter Sixteen ~ White Snake Spear

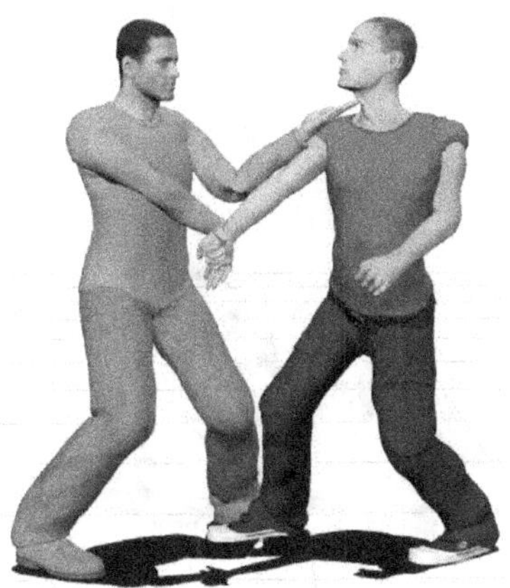

Parry the punch (closing the attack across your body) and spear to the throat (or the axilla). Guide his arm down so you don't jam your fingers into his shoulder.

White Snake Spear (opening)

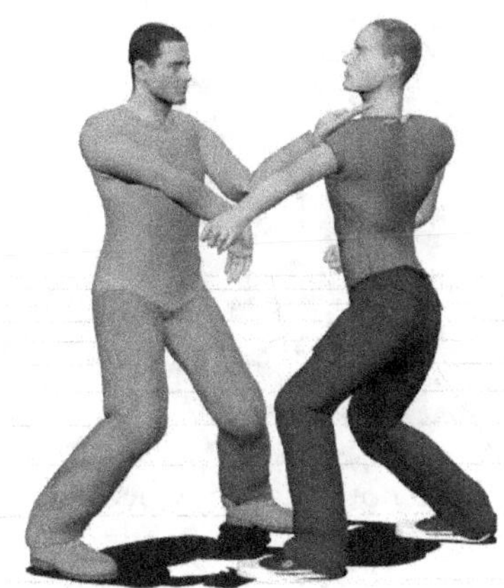

Parry the punch (opening the attack away from your body) and spear to the throat (or the axilla).

White Snake Splitting Arms

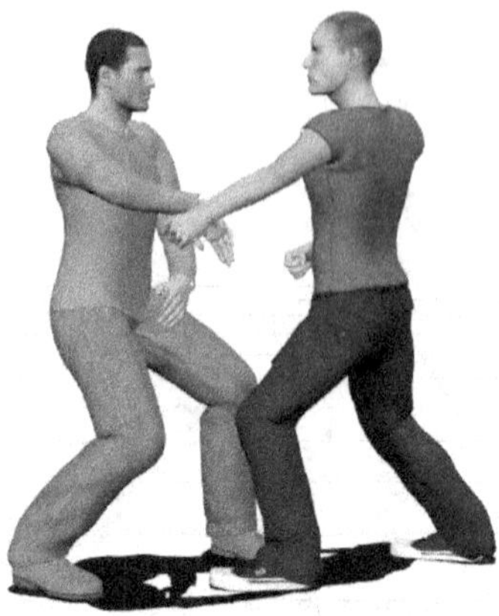

This technique can be used against two strikes in a row, or a simultaneous double strike (two hand push-split the hands and push and pull on them to turn the attacker over). Parry the attacker's first punch outward to the side.

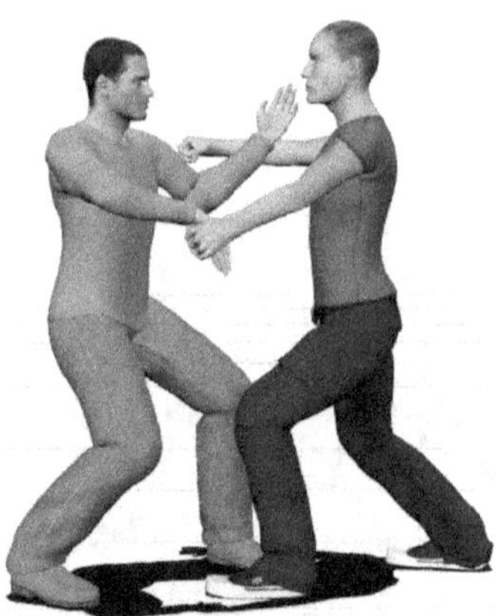

He can retract his punch or not, but block his second strike with a spear transformed into a block. Blocks of this nature should be shooting out from the tan tien, not moving sideways in front of the body.

In the top figure the defender kicks the groin, or the knees. Kicking the back leg under the hip will dislocate the leg and cause extreme pain. It can even break the femoral head (the knob on top of the thigh bone).

In the second picture the defender simply punches the attacker in the throat. One would probably use a half fist to get under the bone of the chin.

In the third picture, my favorite, a thumb into the side of the neck.

Also, most important and something for you to think about…you can bring the left hand down and pull the wrist down, and shoot the right hand in a palm up spear under the attacker's right elbow. You would be doing a White Snake on the other side, and be in a perfect position for using it to arm throw the attacker.

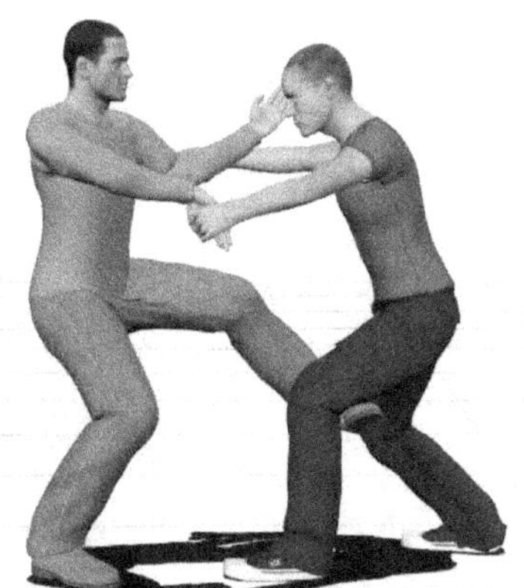

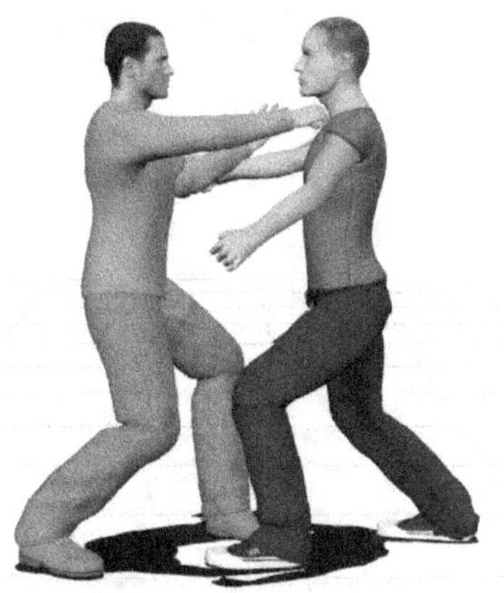

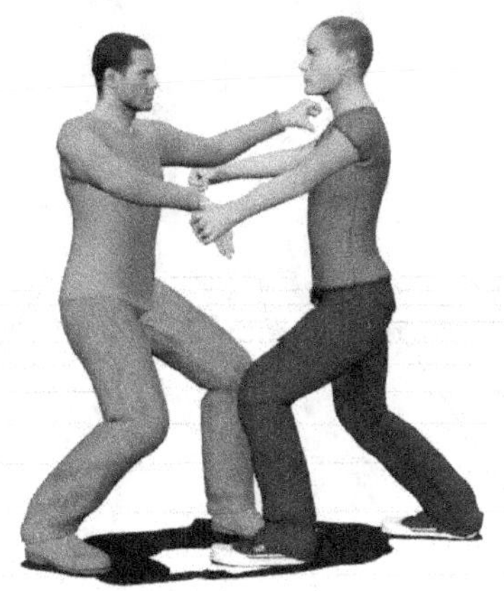

White Snake Splitting

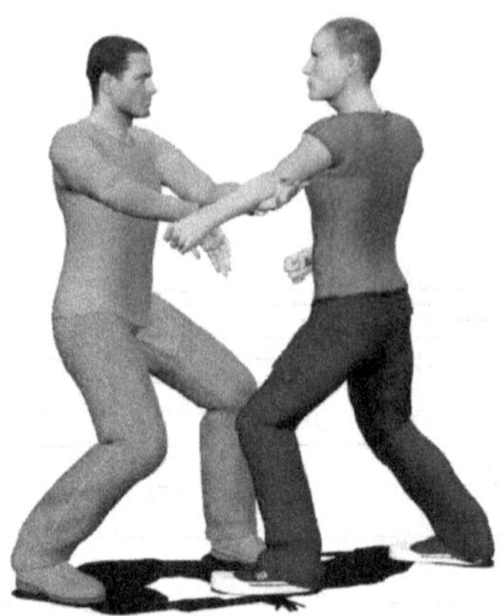

Parry the strike outwards and thrust your palm up spear hand under his elbow.

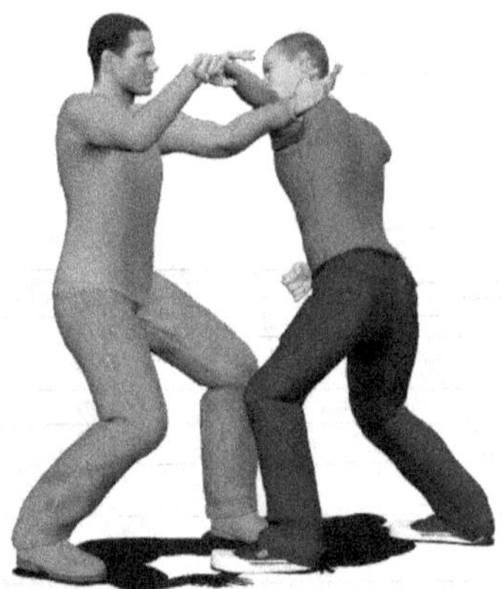

You can grab his wrist, or just use the bar of your forearm, and pull the attacker up and around.

You will have to turn the hips and use the whole body.

You will likely have to step forward with the right foot.

If he wiggles and bends his elbow there are a variety of elbow locks you can slide into, which we will discuss in later techniques.

White Snake from Kang Duk Won

Martial Arts techniques are the same from art to art, but also different, utilize different principles, and show a great variety for interpretations.

Following is a 'White Snake' technique we used to practice in the Kang Duk Won.

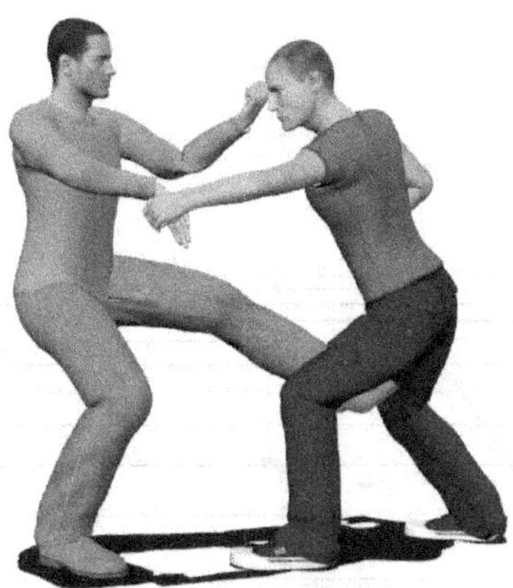

Simultaneously execute a parry, a backfist to the face and a kick to the groin.

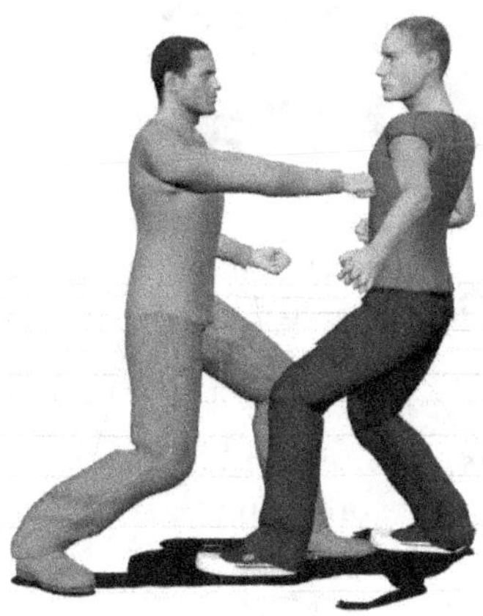

Move in with a full body weight punch to the body. Or a spear to the neck, or a thumb to the side of the neck, or a poke to the eyes, or whatever.

Some people want karate (martial arts) to be polite, but when your life is at stake you must embrace and *enjoy* brutality.

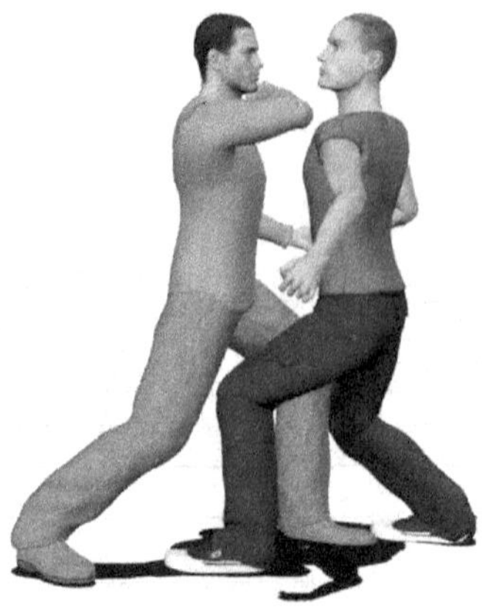

A secondary technique would be to strike with the elbow.

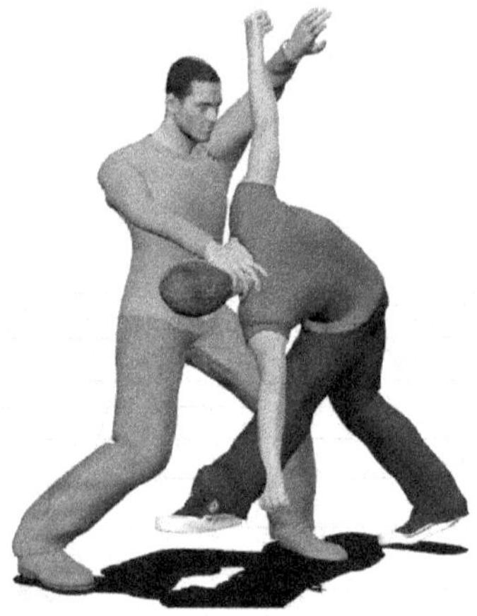

Then push down on the side of the attacker's head as you spiral his right arm up. I refer to this as a vertical arm pin. You can throw him down hard, or find a wrist twist and hold him in a lock.

Some of these techniques may seem a bit busy, but we would practice them until we could make them work. Simply, we worked on them until they worked.

Also, and most important, none of these techniques were posers; you don't do a technique while the attacker waits in position for you to do the technique.

You have to move with, or before, the attacker, and you have to be so polished and harmonious in your movements that your whole body is like sleight of hand to the opponent. That is the essence of making a poser technique into a real technique.

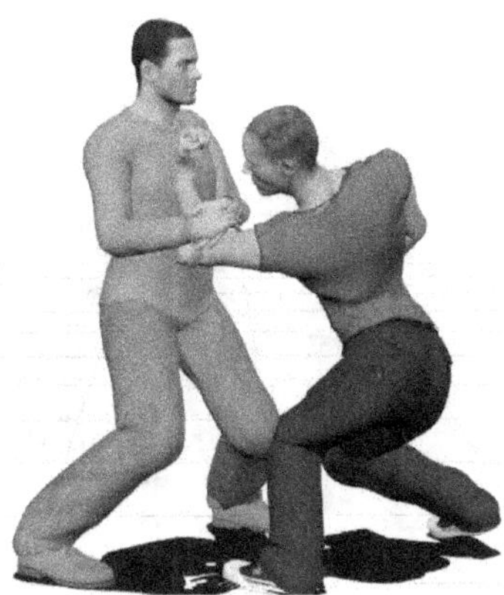

There are many strikes, blocks, locks, throws, that one can develop from the White snake.

Consider the above technique. Can you pull the attacker's elbow to your chest and bend the knees, or simply bow, and cause the attacker to drop to the floor using the White Snake?

Many of the techniques you see her will morph into other techniques, especially as the attacker tries to wiggle and escape. The trick is not to be rigid, but to do these techniques enough times that you can predict what his motions will be, and go with him…right into another technique.

Chapter Seventeen ~ Tiger in a Cave

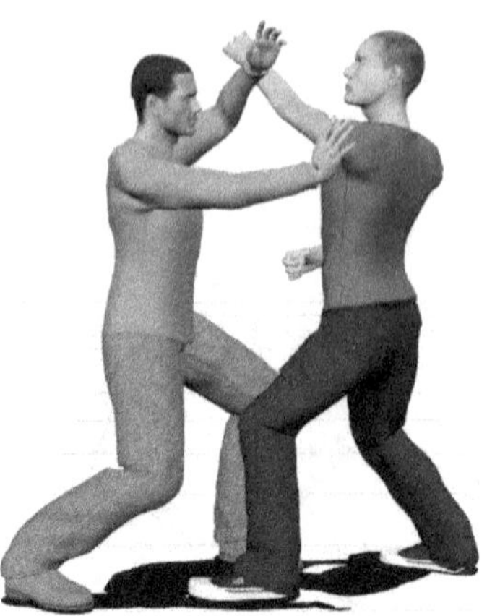

A simple high block with a palm push. A universal technique is one that works on both sides. Whether a person is closing or opening, whether it is the right or the left, it doesn't matter, the technique works.

When you are closing the person, pushing the arm across the person's front to trap their body, the technique looks like this.

Push up on the shoulder and unbalance the attacker. Once he is unbalanced you may follow up with whatever strieks you wish, or even just squat and do a leg takedown, or just kick the leg with yours.

Tiger in a Cave Upper Armlock

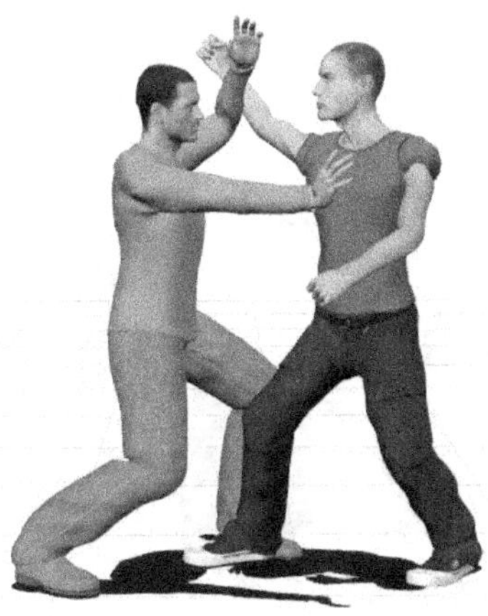

Step forward, jamming the person's attack and forcing his punching arm outwards (opening him).

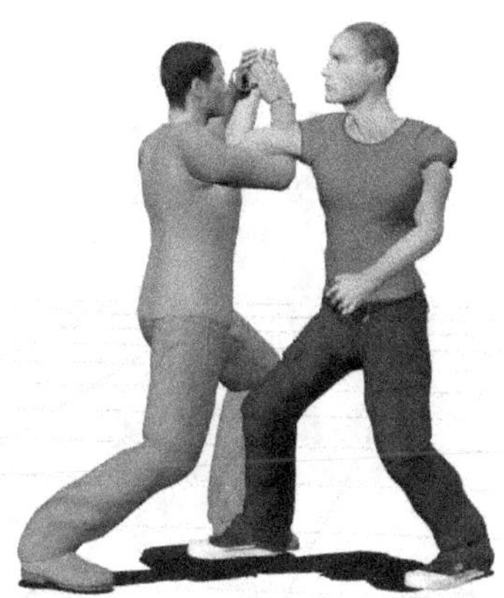

Move forward and angle to the side as you press his right arm back, then slip your right arm under his triceps and up. Clasp both hands and force his arm back to break the elbow.

If he wiggles in an attempt to get out simply turn to the left and break his now straightened out elbow over your shoulder.

White Snake/Tiger in a Cave

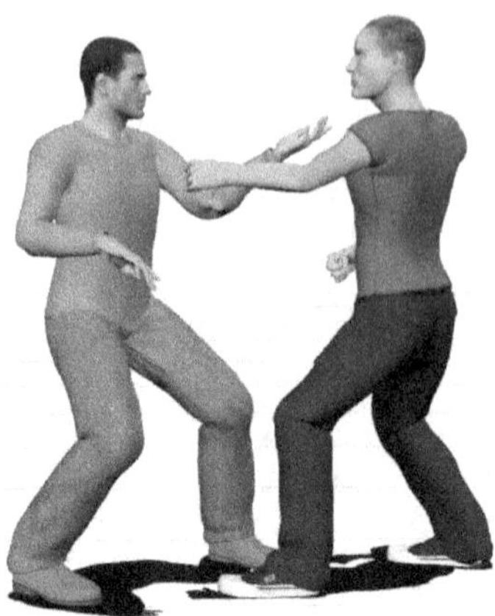

This is a put together of the two techniques, White Snake and Tiger in a Cave.

Execute a left inward block.

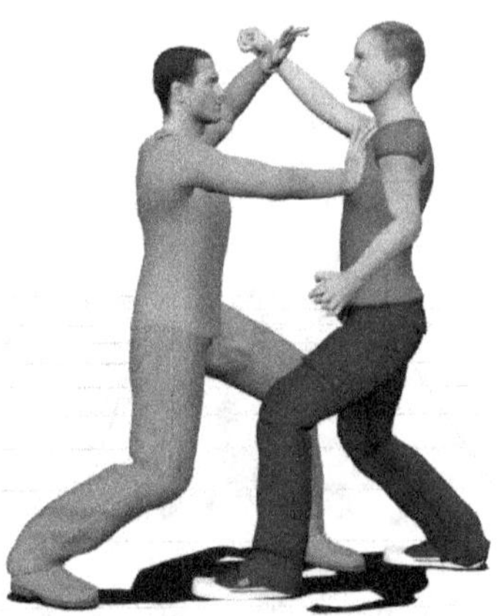

When the attacker comes in with a second punch execute a Tiger in the Cave. Tiger in the Cave will work wonderfully for straight punches, or hook punches. Many martial arts don't deal with hook punches. They train with straight and don't consider that most punches are hooks. Very odd, but understandable considering the technique may have bene developed for weapons.

To use Tiger against a hook punch requires adjustments in footwork and angles.

Chapter Eighteen ~ In Sweep

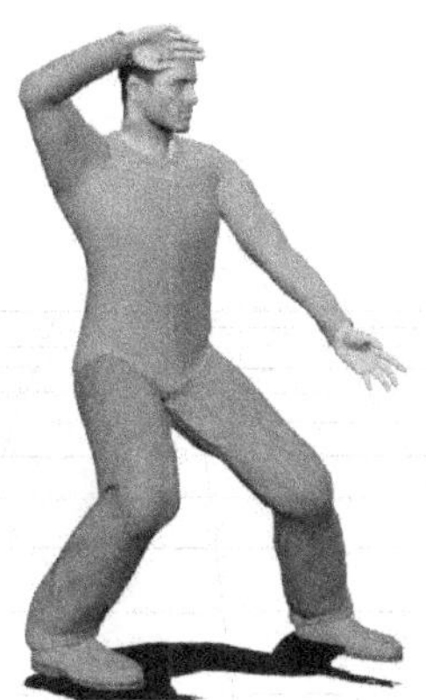

The move between Tiger in the Cave (high block and palm thrust) and Single Whip involves a circling of the arms. This circling goes through the above posture, which I just call 'In Sweep.'

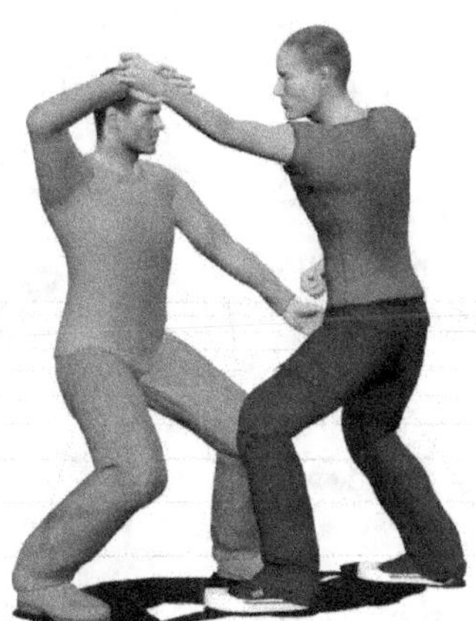

The obvious technique is to step forward, or back, to achieve correct distance. This is the distance at which the attacker thinks he is able to punch you.

As you step you guide the left hand with your right high block. Make sure you turn the hips as the lower hand slaps or grabs him in the groin.

In sweep Out

Another obvious technique is to use this technique for a leg slap, or a leg grab and lift.

In the top picture the defender is slapping the foot outward. This will turn the attacker in so he has to punch with the right hand.

If you scoop the leg and lift the fellow will go down.

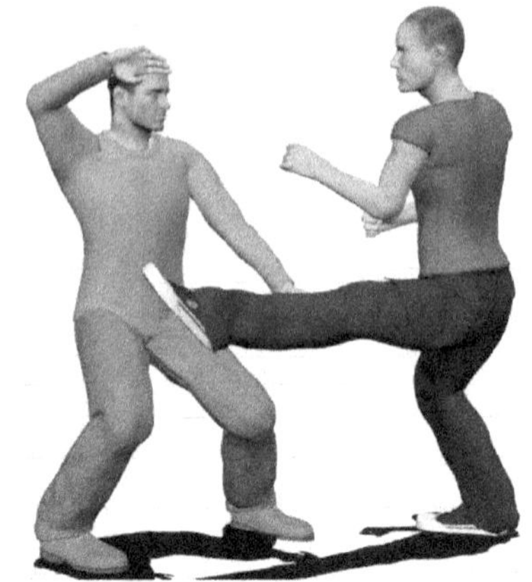

In the middle picture the attacker has thrown a right punch. Don't turn the hips, just align the body and execute a left outward block. By not turning the hips you ground, let the energy run through the body, and the attacker simply runs into your unbendable arm.

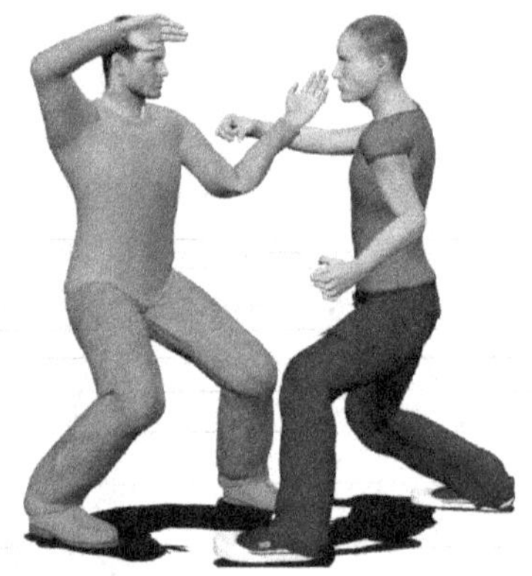

In the bottom picture the form would demand a beak strike (grouped fingers). I have never been a believer in the beak, I think the grouped fingers indicates a grab. So I opt to execute a snapping palm. The beak starts the motion, but the palm snaps down to the top of the forehead.

One could also chop the collar bone, poke the eyes (beak?), etc.

One could also truncate the technique by executing a left palm after the second picture.

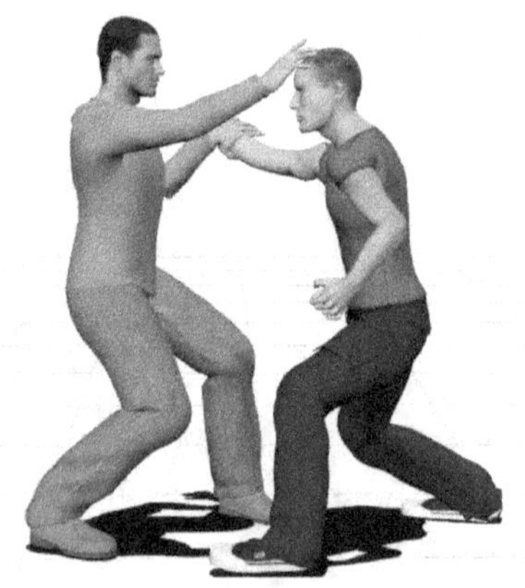

Chapter Nineteen ~ Single Whip

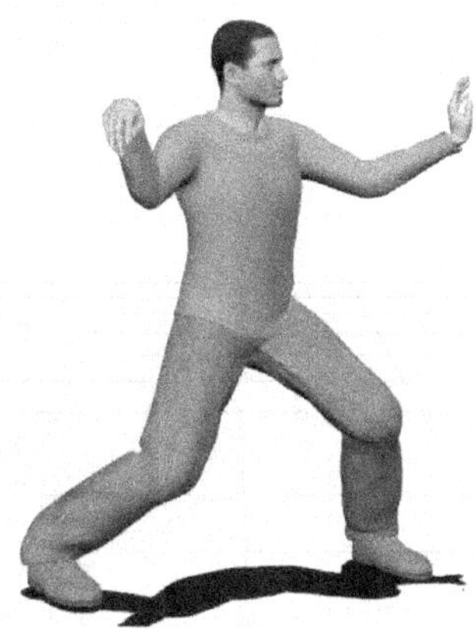

There are a host of things wrong with Single Whip, yet it has become somewhat iconic when referring to Tai Chi Chuan.

So, do you push his chest and poke a beak at a pressure point on his very long wrist?

Do you hold the tip of a spear and reach in to palm strike him?

The posture is wrong, you see.

So, how do we fix it, how do we assume a better example of the ten arm positions, how do we make it functional in combat?

Very and incredibly easy: add a slap grab.

Single Whip Slap/Grab

Slap the punch.

The other arm circles under and around to grip the wrist.

Pull the wrist, move forward and palm strike the chest.

Voila! Single Whip working.

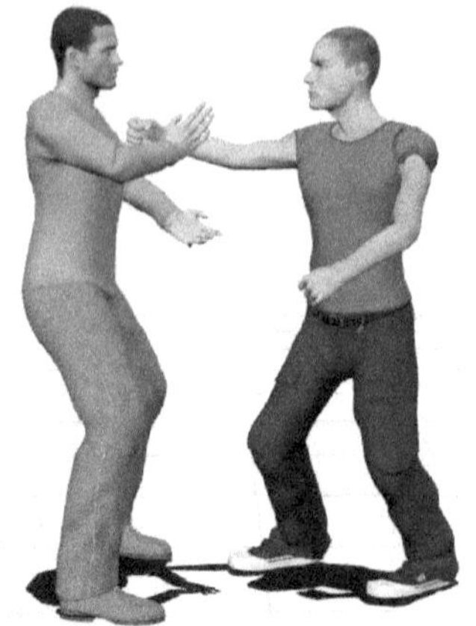

People almost never understand the value of a. slap, as in the slap/grab.

If a fly was bugging you you wouldn't execute a massive power high bock. You simply slap the bugger.

A punch is nothing but a fly to somebody who has practiced enough.

10,000 times is enough, especially considering that the Chinese considered 10,000 to represent 'forever.'

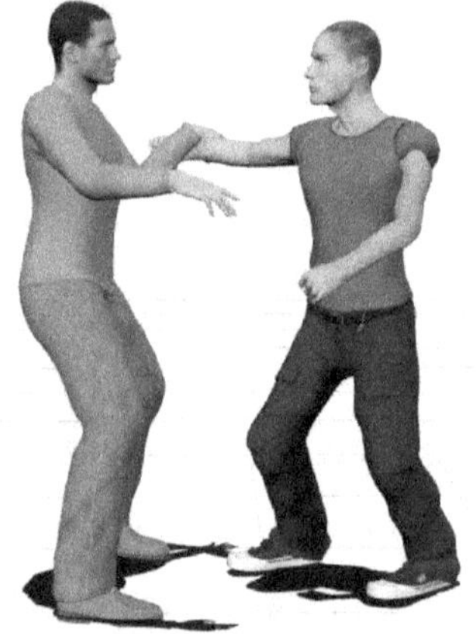

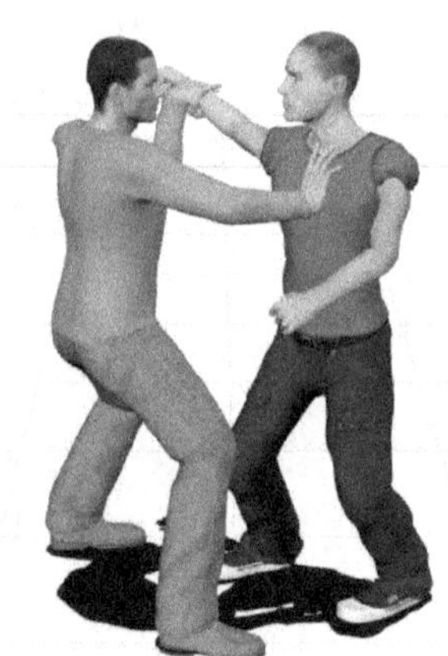

Single Whip Arm Splitting

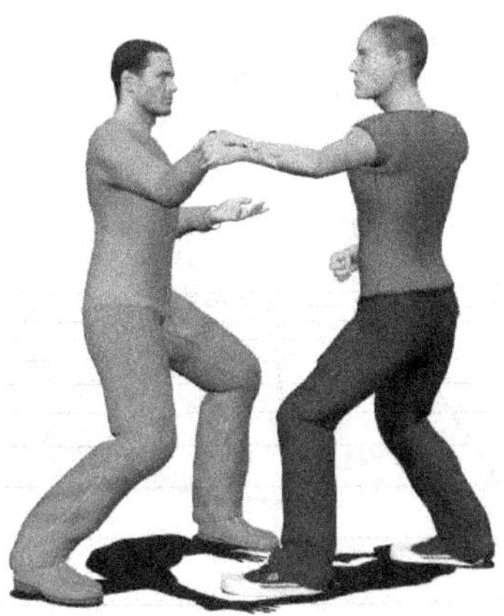

Step slightly to the side and catch the attacker's punch. Hold it if you can, or this is useful if he just keeps pressing.

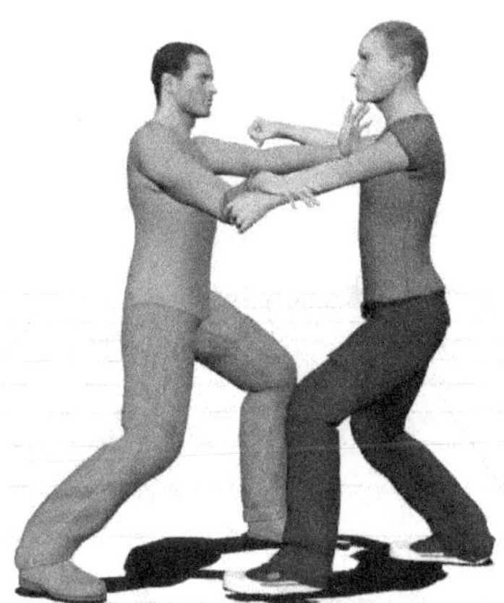

When he throws the second punch move forward and palm strike the biceps.

You can end the technique and cause good pain if you just punch the bicep.

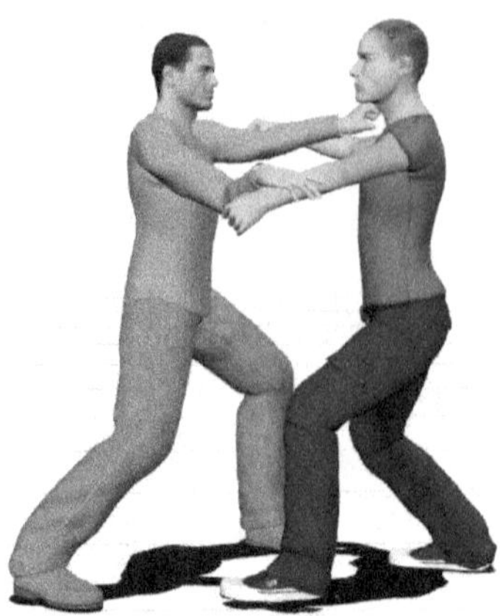

You can punch or kick. Good targets include a half fist to the throat or a spear to the eyes.

My favorite is a simple thumb to the side of the neck. I suggest you practice doing push ups on your thumbs for a while before attempting to do this.

I have also found there are sensitive areas between the muscles on the side of the biceps, and on the crown of the biceps.

This is a tricky technique that require practice, but the essence is to watch the person's body, not his arms. All strikes emanate from the tan tien, the closer your observation gets to the tan tien, and this simply means earlier on the body (the dip of the shoulders, the movement of his back, the focus of his eyes, etc.)

Chapter Twenty ~ Inverted Pole Position

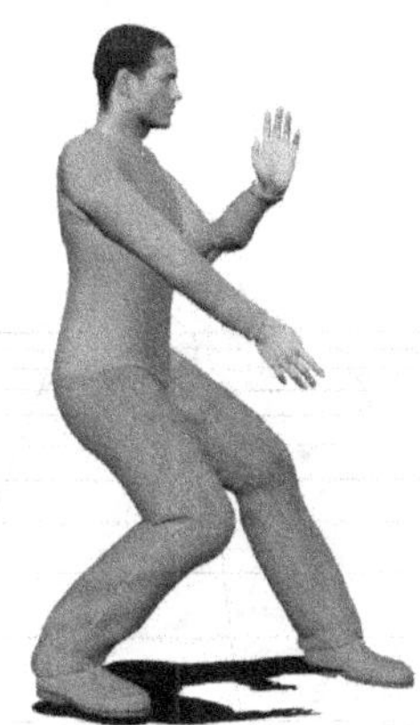

From Single Whip one must retreat as he is over committed. This involves a twisting of the body as you move it into a back stance.

I call this the Inverted Pole Position. The standard Pole Position would have the front hand on the bottom, the rear hand on the top.

I call it the pole position because you stand as if you are holding a staff vertical in front of you.

Normally I don't like crossing the body to block. We actually avoid this like the plague when doing the Lop Sau (circling hands) drill.

Because of the necessity of the form protecting oneself with a twist, we do it here.

You will see, in the next technique, how this move is used to feed into Lop Sau.

You should be exploring every technique with Lop Sau.

How can you utilize White Cran with Lop Sau?

How can you adapt Single Whip inside of Lop Sau.

Inverted Pole Position for Kick

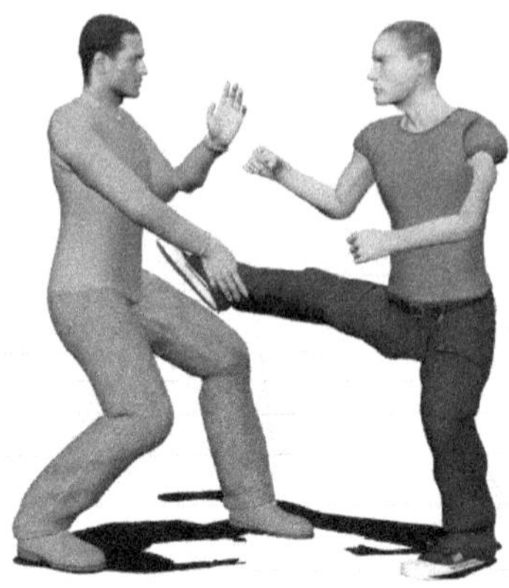

When the attacker kicks you slap down with the palm, guiding his foot outward so he will have to punch with the left hand.

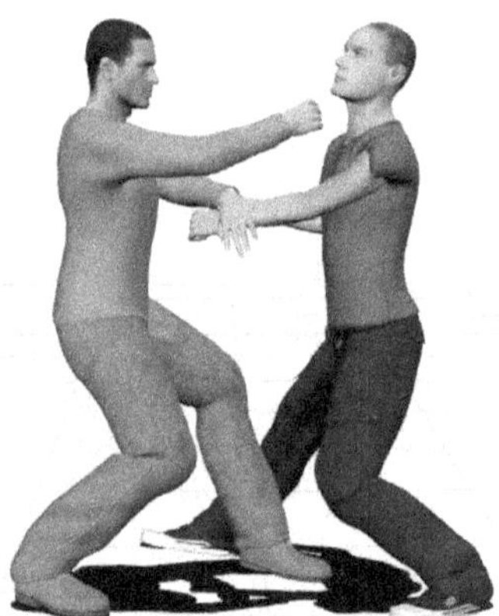

When the attacker punches roll the left hand down on his punch, smothering it as you roll your own punch over and into his face.

Shuffle forward to add body weight to the strike; strike with your whole body weight.

I always prefer guiding a foot, rather than executing a hard low block. Don't block a larger body part with your smaller body part, if possible, and the technique segues directly into rolling hands.

Chapter Twenty-One ~ White Crane Strike or Split

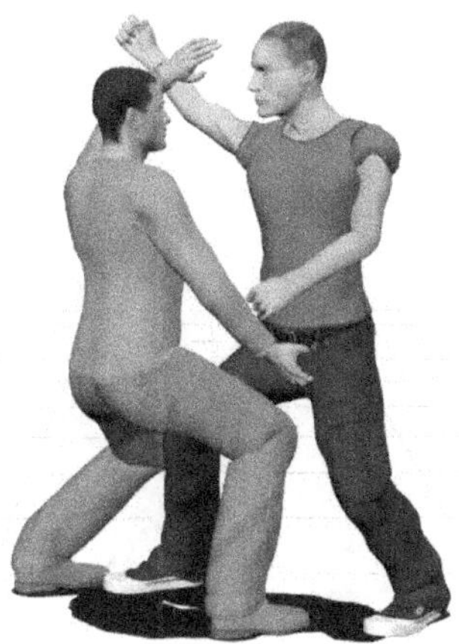

White Crane can be done in a variety of ways, but does require some adjustment. Just remember that it is one of the basic arm positions. the basic arm positions (listed earlier in the book) are those positions which create the most energy with the least work.

In the above example I've got the posture backwards from the traditional, but one arm is down and one arm is up. Classic, but unorthodox White Crane.

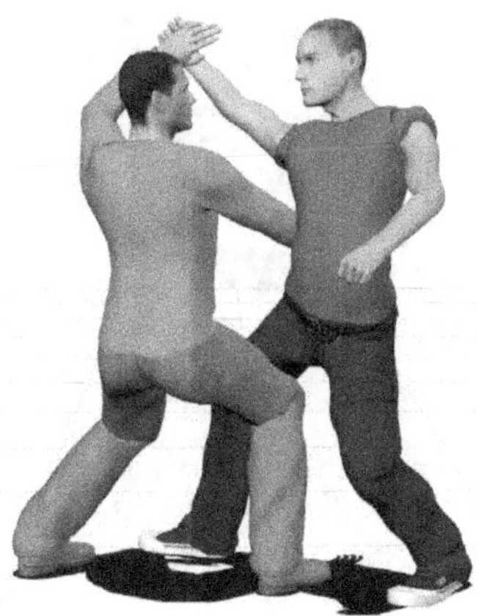

If you angle the body differently you can forget about the groin and go deeper, extend your arm behind the attacker and split him.

White Crane Strike or Split (2)

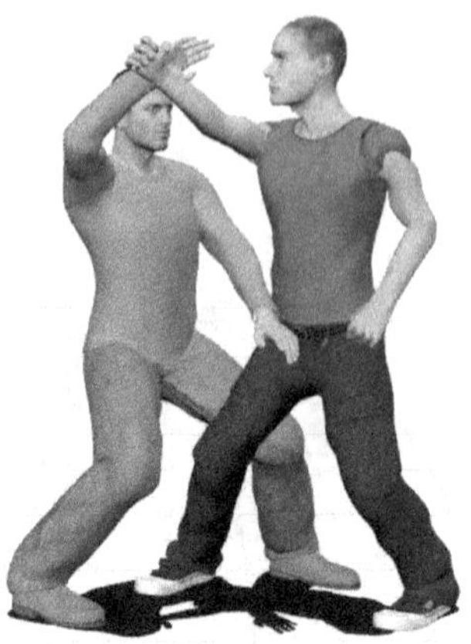

Another example of guiding the strike while slapping the groin. One could easily grab the leg and lift the opponent to throw.

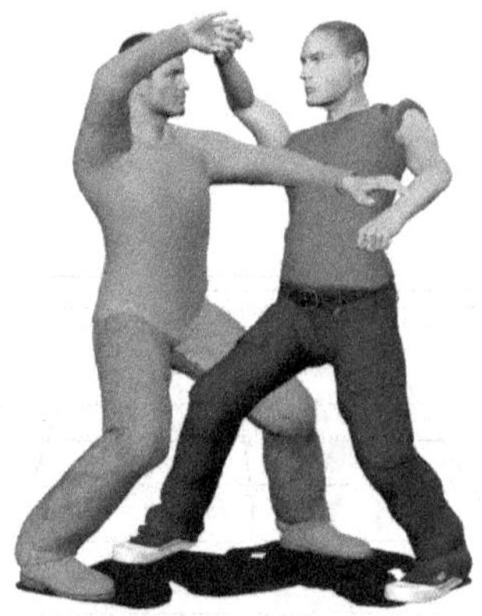

Raising the arm results in a split.

People don't seem to understand the importance of classical postures. They want to focus on punching and kicking. Nothing wrong with destruction, but the true art is in control. The classic postures lean to control.

White Crane for Kick

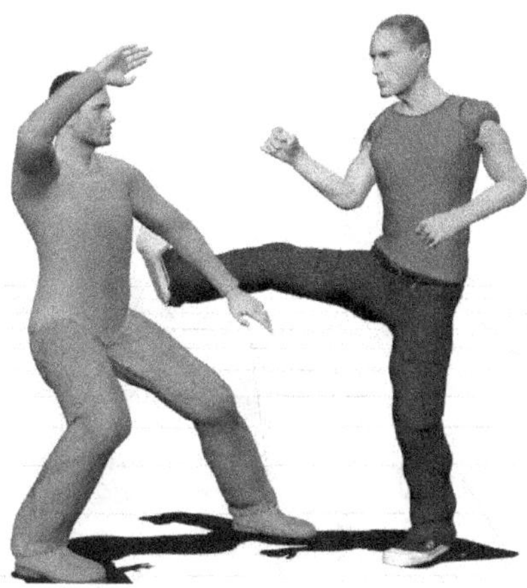

Execute a What Crane low block, the high hand doesn't do anything but circle around.

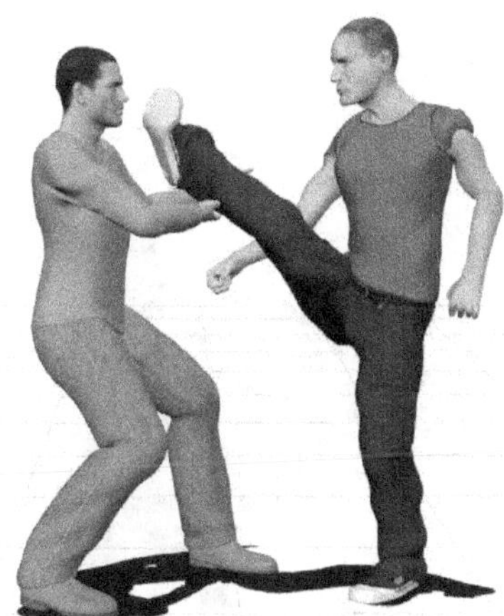

Snake the low block under the kick and lift, the right hand can help lift. When I first learned this I didn't have the the strength to lift, so I would get low and jam the leg into the crotch of my arm and lift with my legs.

If he's flexible and doesn't turn into a side position (very common when they run out of flexibility) you can kick or sweep his support leg.

Chapter Twenty-Two ~ Punch Under

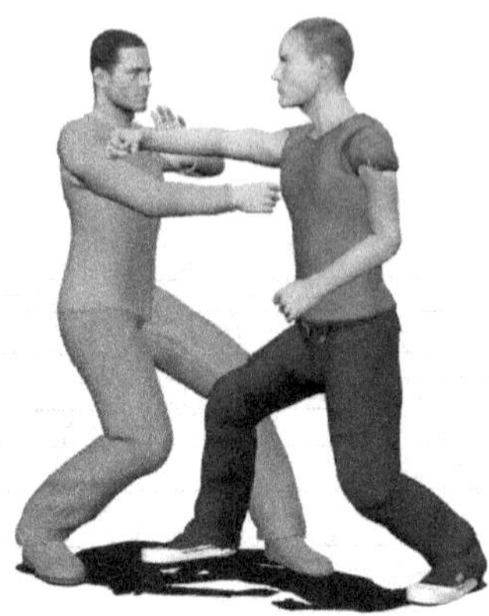

Punch Under demonstrates how techniques roll from one to another smoothly and easily.

The defender steps slightly to the side and evades the punch, and guides the punch, and punches to the body,

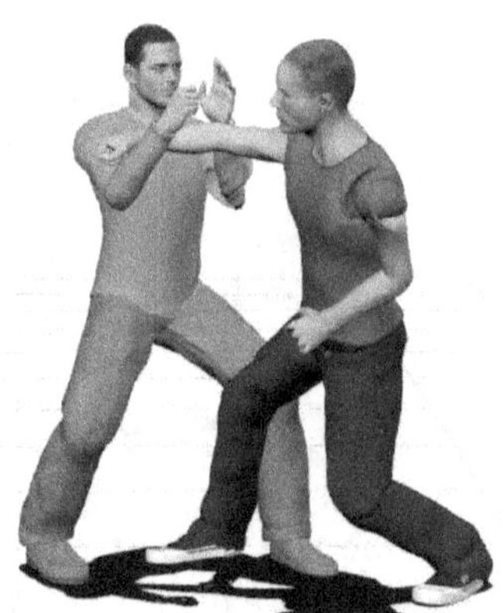

The defender can simply twist the hips and break the elbow, or go into an arm bar or an elbow roll.

Refer back to Roll back to see how the technique can progress into elbow spikes and splits.

Punch Under Elbow Drop

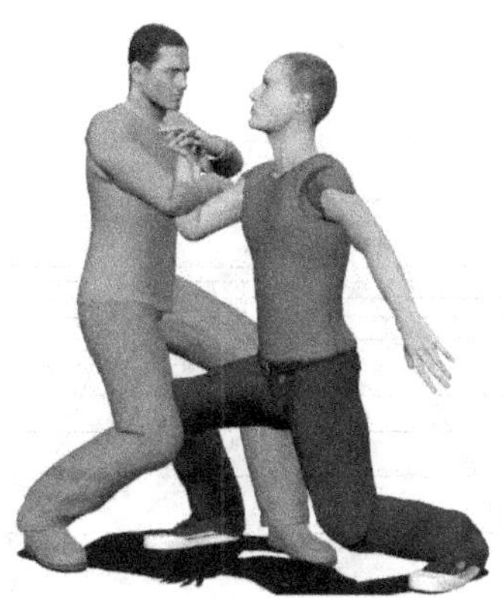

OR…from the punch under (first photo last page) one can wrap the left arm over the crotch of the elbow, hug the arm and pull down. Note that there is a wrist twist in the above picture.

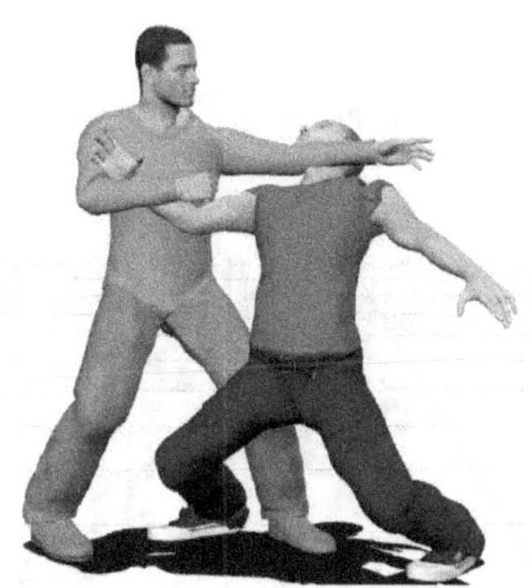

When the attacker goes down step and twist and split him over your leg with an arm extended to his throat.

This is directly from Monkey Boxing.

Chapter Twenty-Three ~ Pole Position

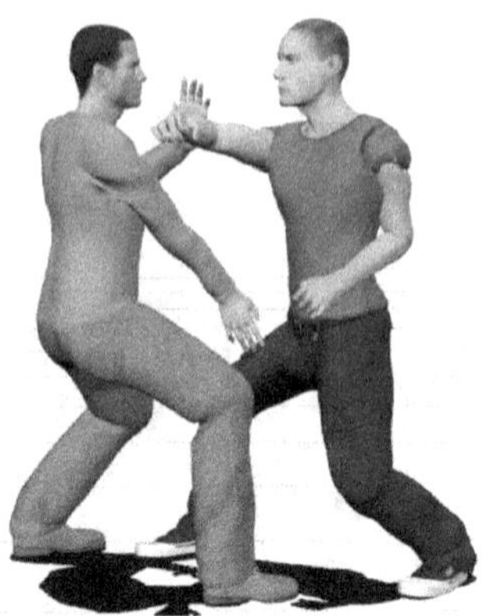

Whenever somebody is doing Pole Position they should be looking to enter Lop Sau. Yes, you can go into locks, but the main emphasis is to teach the student how to take control of an attack.

The defender slaps the punch.

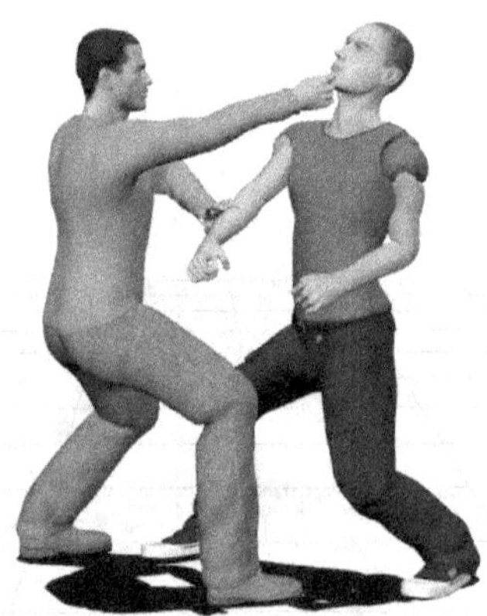

The defender smothers the punch and shuffles forward to roll the fist and strike the face.

One must learn to roll effectively, figuring out which hand should be in the superior position so that he doesn't trap his own hands.

Pole Position

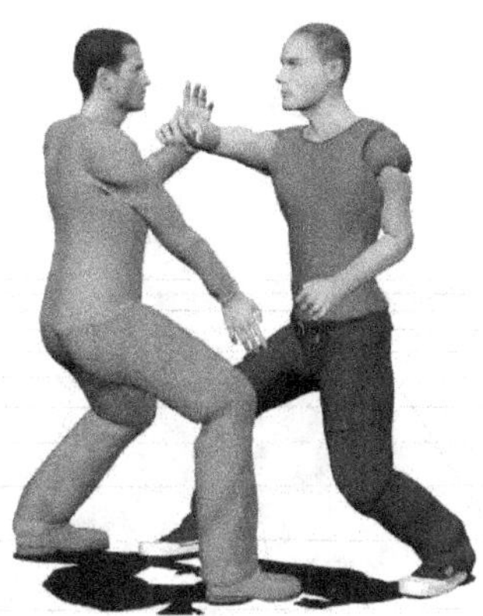

Slap the fist to close the attacker.

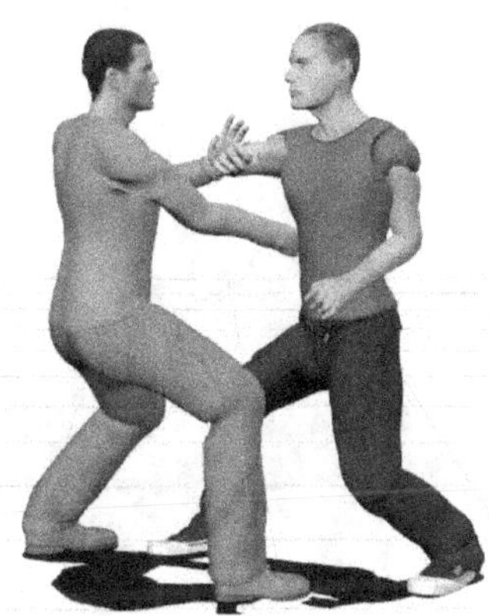

Press his arm inward so he can't lower it for a block. and execute a punch or a backfist to the body.

I'm not fond of back fists. They don't lend themselves to the full body weight strikes that I like. However, because this position is sometimes too awkward for power punches, if you're fast enough you can slap a backfist into his ribs and do some serious damage.

You can also wrap the arms, or execute other other techniques.

Chapter Twenty-Four ~ Ward Off

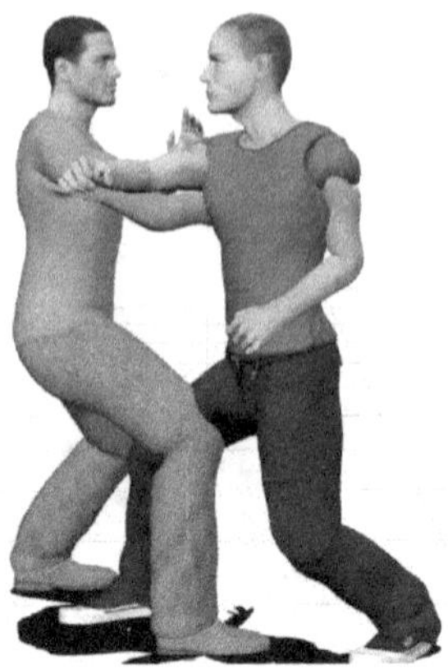

To execute this technique one has to slap the punch aside and assume a position close tot he opponent, with the rounded right hand *touching the opponent's body.*

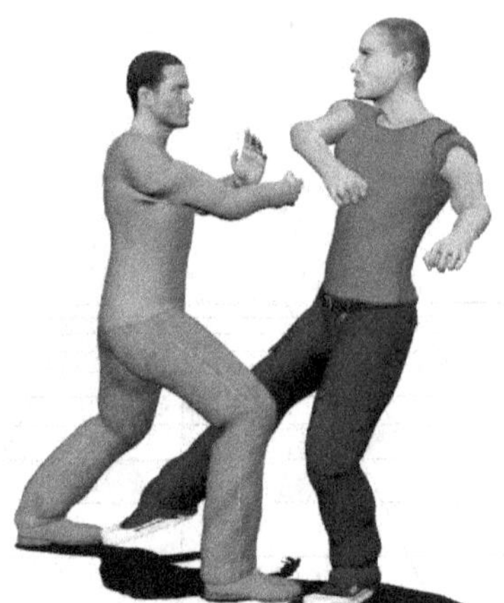

Push with the legs, uprooting the opponent and sending him 12 to 20 feet.

One can do things like wrapping the arm and pulling down, elbow strikes, and moving in with a horse stance to split his body.

Ward Off Splitting

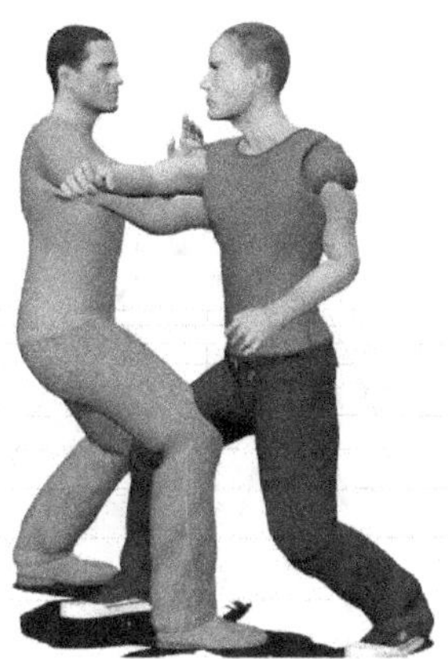

Slap the hand and move into the opponent.

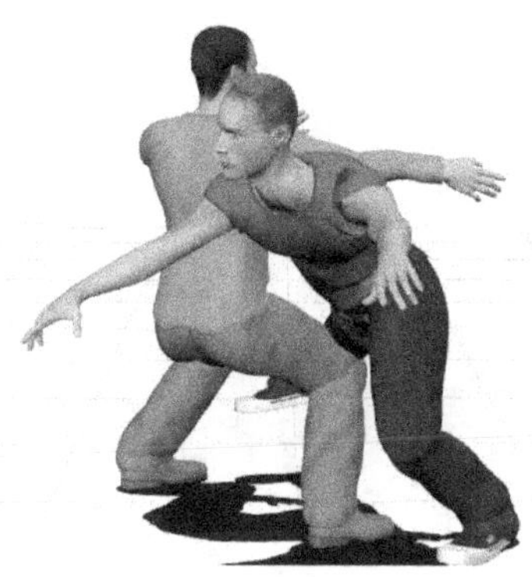

Snug the foot behind the attacker's front foot as you assume a horse stance. Extend the right arm across his lower back.

KEEP BOTH FEET FLAT! DO NOT LIFT YOUR HEEL!

I call this 'Tripping the Tiger' in Monkey Boxing.

These techniques are simple, yet require finesse to work properly. but, as I have said, the art is about control, not force or destruction.

You will actually see these techniques time and again, sometimes with different entries, sometimes in different combination.

Do not think, 'Oh, I know this one.' Instead, just practice it as if you don't know it, and need ten thousand repetitions.

Remember this one phrase, which is one of the most important in all of the martial arts:

There are no secret techniques,

there are just better basics!

Chapter Twenty-Five

Matrixing Techniques

Usually, when you create a matrix for an art, it is best to keep it simple. For instance, here is a basic matrix for the four basic karate blocks.

	Lo	Hi	In	Out
Lo	Lo/Lo	Lo/Hi	Lo/In	Lo/Out
Hi	Hi/Lo	Hi/Hi	Hi/In	Hi/Out
In	In/Lo	In/Hi	In/In	In/Out
Out	Out/Lo	Out/Hi	Out/In	Out/Out

One uses one one block for the basic technique, then combines it with the other blocks. This is much better than just making a list, as it gives a person the complete picture of what they are doing.

When doing the matrix for the Advanced Nine Square Diagram techniques, however, I have used 8 techniques. You can make the number of techniques more or less as you wish.

You can make a matrix with eight boxes across and twelve boxes down, but it is actually simpler to just make eight lists.

On the following page are the first two lists so you will understand we are just taking one technique for the base, then just combining with the others.

ROLL BACK AS THE BASE TECHNIQUE

1. Roll Back/Roll Back

2. Roll Back/Brush Knee

3. Roll Back/White Snake

4. Roll Back/Tiger in Cave

5. Roll Back/Single Whip

6. Roll Back/White Crane

7. Roll Back/Punch Under

8. Roll Back/Ward Off

BRUSH KNEE AS THE BASE TECHNIQUE

Brush Knee/Roll Back

Brush Knee/Brush Knee

Brush Knee/White Snake

Brush Knee/Tiger in Cave

Brush Knee/Single Whip

Brush Knee/White Crane

Brush Knee/Punch Under

Brush Knee/Ward Off

The next list would have the White Snake as the base technique.

Remember, these are not basics, they are applying the Ten Arm Positions through the most useful of martial arts postures.

Combine the techniques as you wish. Remember that you can enter the techniques from different positions, reverse the arm motions, and so on.

It is not the direction of the legs/arms/body into the postures that is important. It is important to find the positions that use the least energy.

section four

Freestyle

You must work to make it work.

Chapter Twenty-Sex

Lop Sau

I learned Sticky Hands (from Wing Chun Kung Fu) while at the Kang Duk Won. Bob Babich, the instructor, taught it after one had their black belt. I got the idea that he felt it would be too difficult for beginners, or even people below black belt, to learn.

Years later I learned Pushing Hands (from Tai Chi Chuan). Because I was grounded in solid, functional, workable basics, and because I was conversant with the principle of emptying the arms in Sticky Hands, I was able to make it work.

Years after that I was introduced to arm pounding (Indonesian arts, I believe), and I remembered reading about an exercise called Lop Sau, which means 'Circling hands.'

I learned everything in a backward sequence, so when I looked at Lop Sau I could see how incomplete it was.

People used it for conditioning, or some other reason.

But as I delved into it I saw endless applications, how the thing could be made more whole, and so on.

I developed Lop Sau, with the six basic moves, as you will see it in the coming pages.

I learned how to combine it with other methods of freestyle according to the distances involved.

I eventually developed the grab arts that were core to the arts, and which were easily learned and even applicable to actual combat.

Six techniques, endless combinations, topped off with the various grab arts.

If you have mastered Lop Sau you can defeat any attacker, step into the ring, and are totally protected.

Seeking violence, or glory, however, is a very short-sighted view when it comes to the enlightening aspects of the drill.

1st Lop Sau Technique

ROLLING THE FIST

The first technique is a simple rolling of the fists, smacking the front fist into the palm of the attacker.

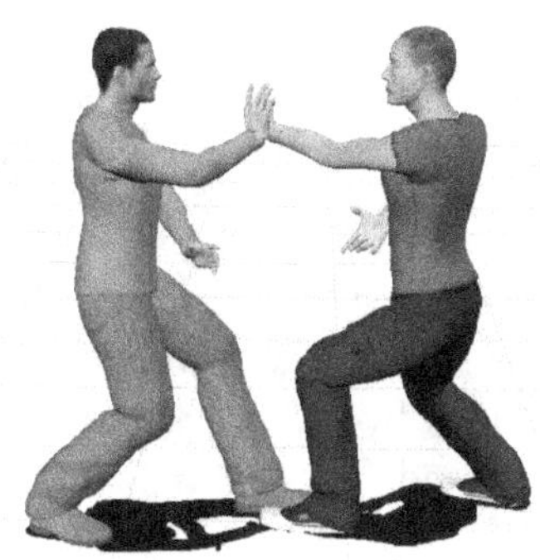

The fist circles in front of the body like a slow buzz saw, which can speed up into a blast of over riding, circling fists, driving down on the attacker's arms as you penetrate his defenses.

You will not that the arms go through the Pole Position. From the Pole Position one can enter the other postures, or simply set one up for attacking (countering.

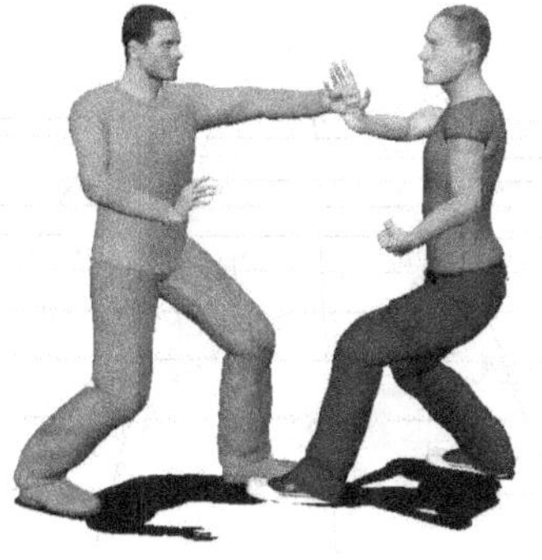

The fist that is hitting the opponent's palm is a back fist in the drill, in reality it is a straight jab to the face.

Shuffling forward as one does this adds body weight, and the jab can become as powerful as a full powered strike with the rear hand.

I have used the images from a. previous book, but have changed the descriptions to better simplify instructions and describe deviations.

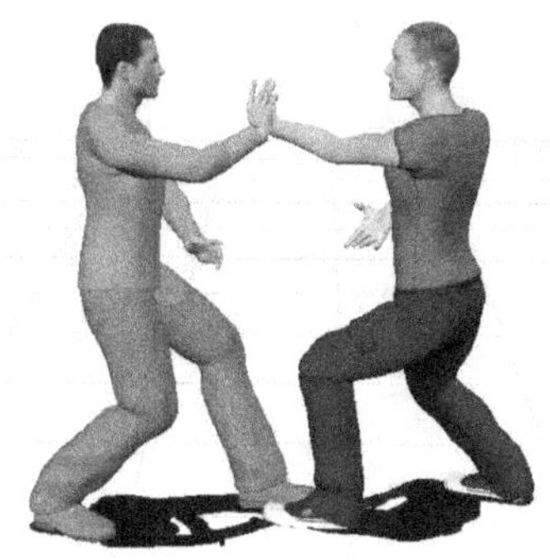

2nd Lop Sau Technique

FRONT HAND HOOK PUNCH

In the second technique the attacker throws a round punch with the front hand. The defender executes a high block.

This exposes the body and the partner throws a body punch, which is deflected by a forearm block with the front hand.

The forearm block is part of the Lop Sau circle of the hands.

The upper block in the beginning is directly from the Tiger in the Cave.

Practice the technique, Tiger in the Cave. Practice Lop Sau until you are fairly competent, then see if you can make Tioger in a Cave work as either the attack or the defense.

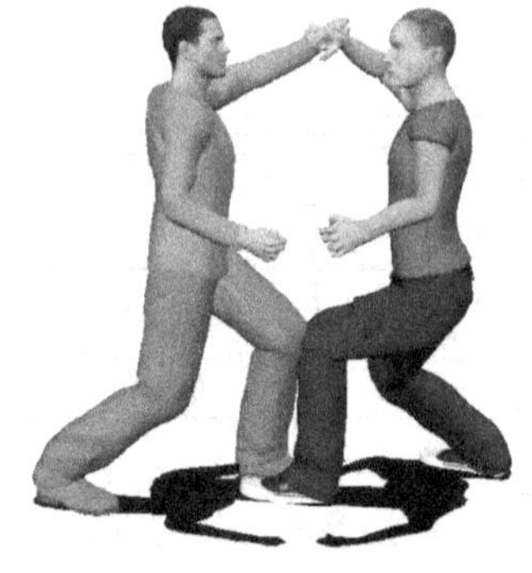

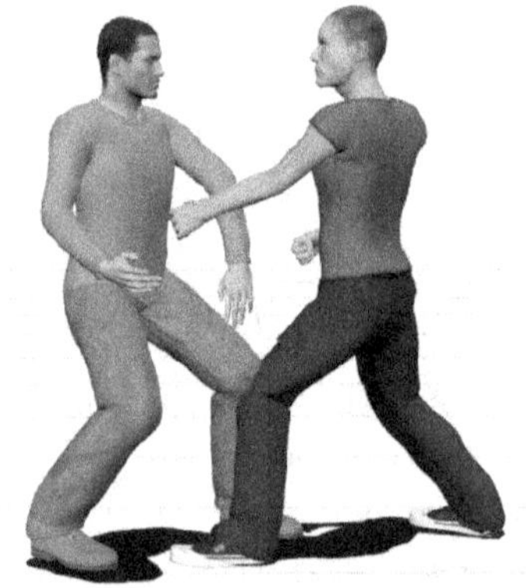

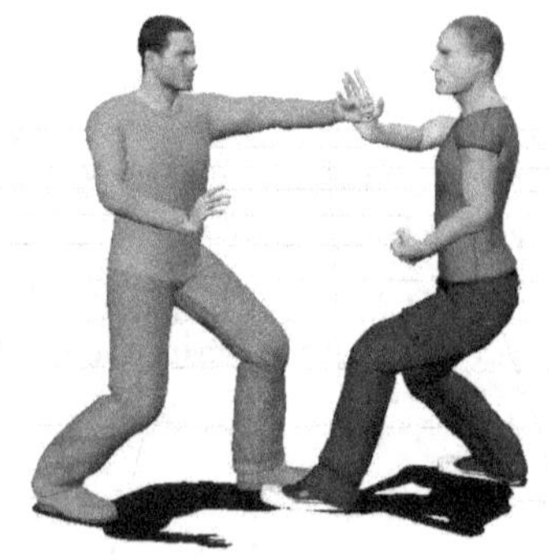

3rd Lop Sau Technique

REAR HAND HOOK PUNCH

The third technique is a hook punch with the rear hand. The defender executes a high block, then counters with a punch to the belly.

The attacker executes a forearm block with the front hand and circles back into the Lop Sau drill with a backfist.

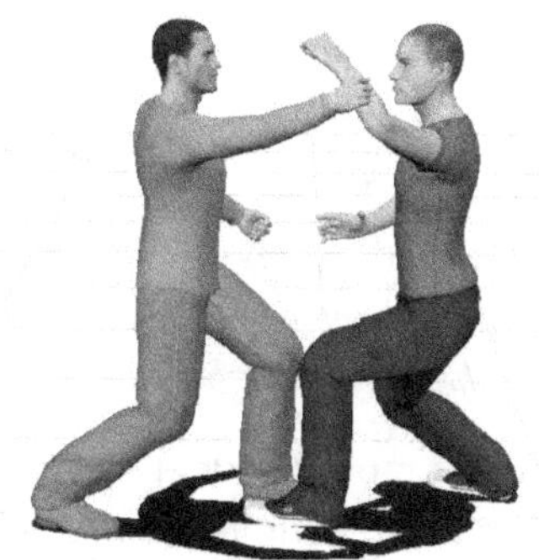

One can see the inverted Pole Position, or the low hand from the inverted white Crane posture.

If you can see these simple connections the techniques will make sense and be expandable to freestyle and realistic combat.

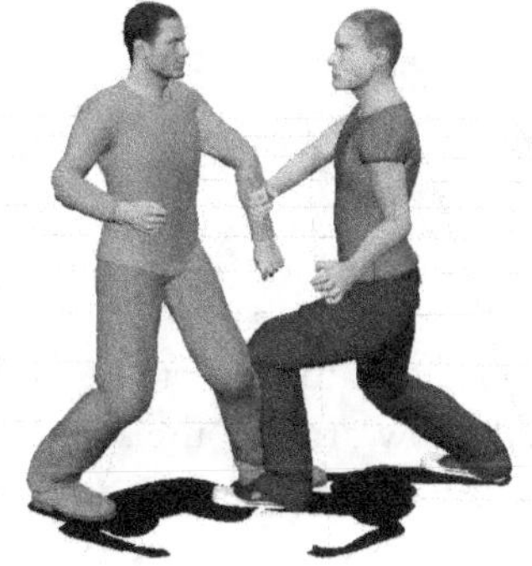

One of the most difficult things is to get the student to attack. He is sort of brain frozen and can only react to the teacher's attacks.

Making the student attack, having him do attacks on beginning students (once he has advanced a bit) will put him at a point of cause. I would hold up any promotion until this simple fact, being able to attack with Lop Sau, is understood and able to be done.

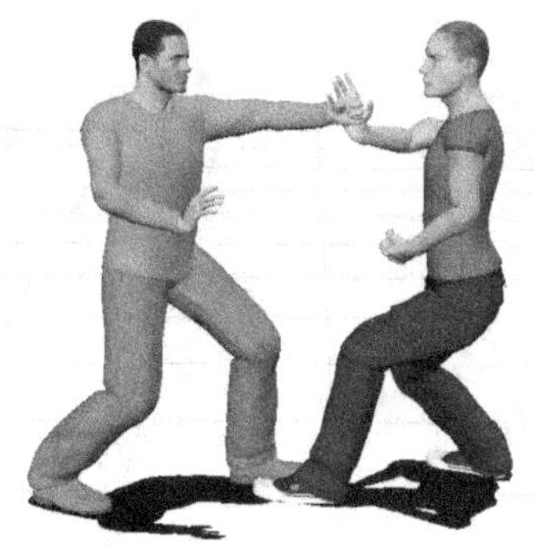

4th Lop Sau Technique

SLAPPING THE FRONT KICK

The fourth technique is using the circling of the hands to slap a front kick outwards, and to continue the circle of the hands to a backfist.

Students always want to use hard, low blocks to defend themselves. Nothing wrong with a good, hard low block, *once the student has properly conditioned his arms through arm bashing drills!*

But it is more efficient to guide a kick, rather than simply smash your arm into it.

Guiding is a higher art, it depends on the student's ability to see what is coming, and it sets up the attacker for the counter.

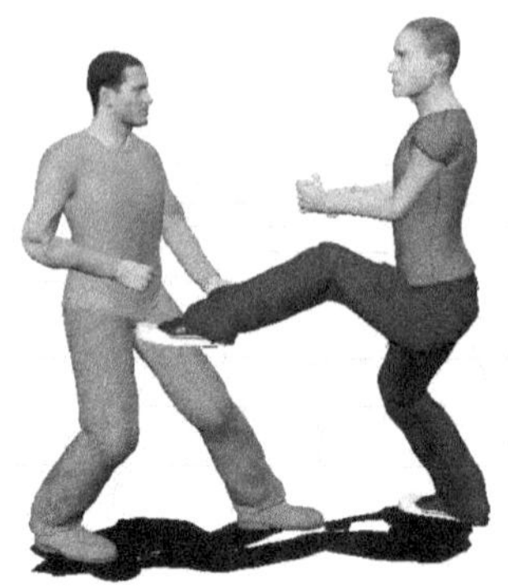

You can see the inverted Pole Position, or the low arm of the Inverted White Crane in this move.

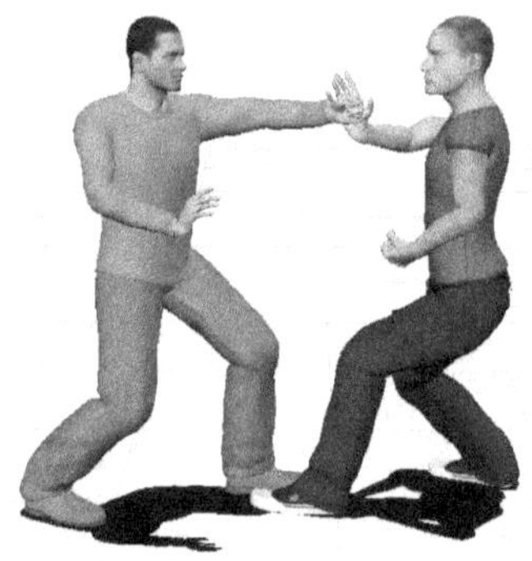

5th Lop Sau Technique

CHANGING SIDES

The fifth technique is to change sides. Instead of stopping the attack with the back hand, guide it with the front hand.

The essence of the move is to synchronize the backward motion of the hand with pulling the front foot back, and to synchronize the stepping forward of the other foot with the attack of the other hand.

When you do this the beginning student will always block with the wrong hand with a high block.

This not only makes the student predictable, but leads into a rolling elbow lock/takedown.

This technique uses the slap of the Slap/Grab move.

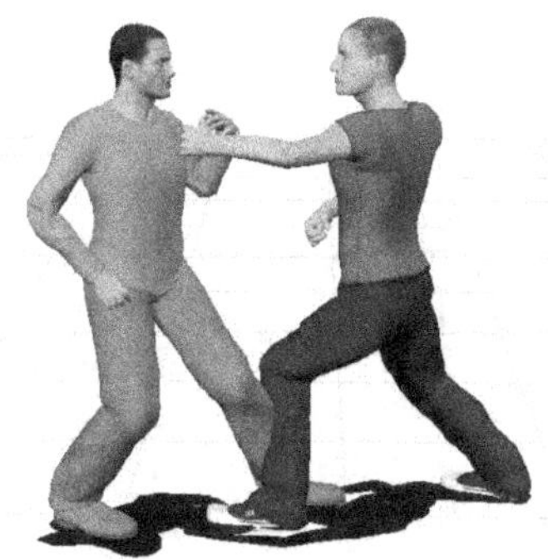

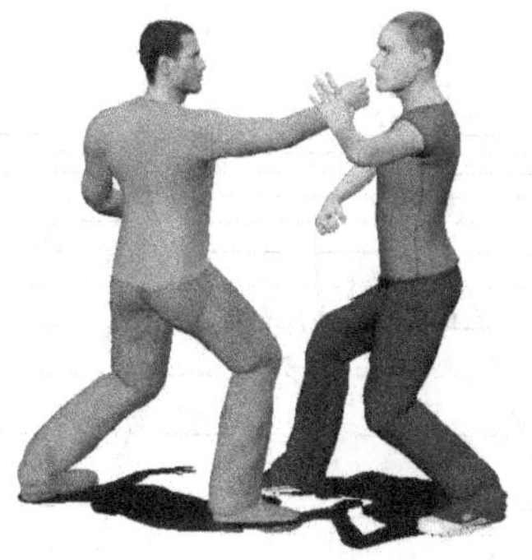

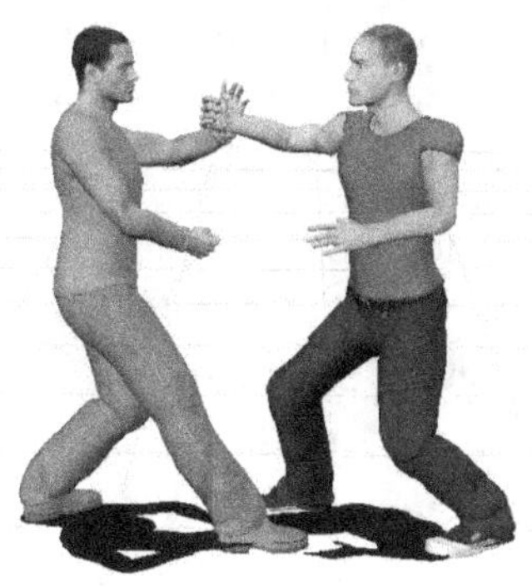

6th Lop Sau Technique

CHANGING WITH A KICK

The sixth technique is to do a change, using the hand techniques of the fifth technique, but instead of punching, doing a kick.

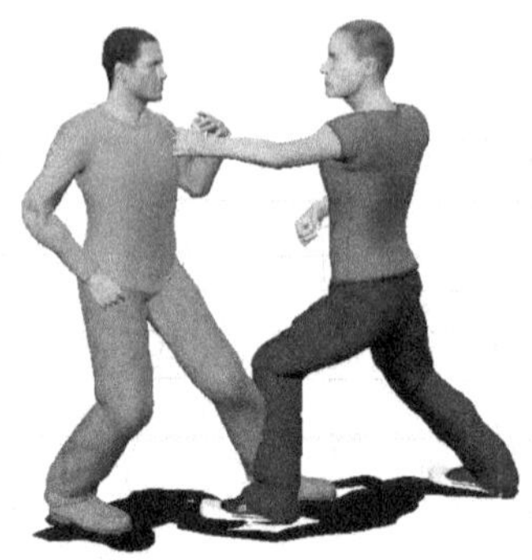

The student will almost always end up doing a hard low block.

If you have conditioned your legs through endless bashing drills you can simply break his arm with your kick.

And if he does do a low block it means he hasn't changed to match you, and you will have a positional advantage. Since he is used to fighting on one side, and you understand the position, you can simply charge in and close him up and run over him.

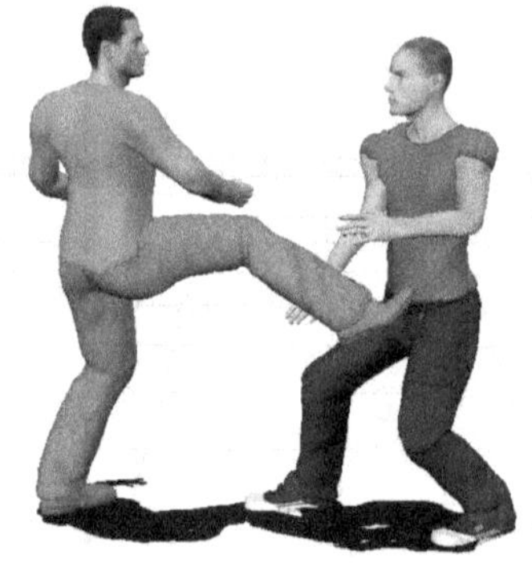

If you hold to the Lop Sau sequence you will wear the other person down, for people have a difficult time repeating simple moves.

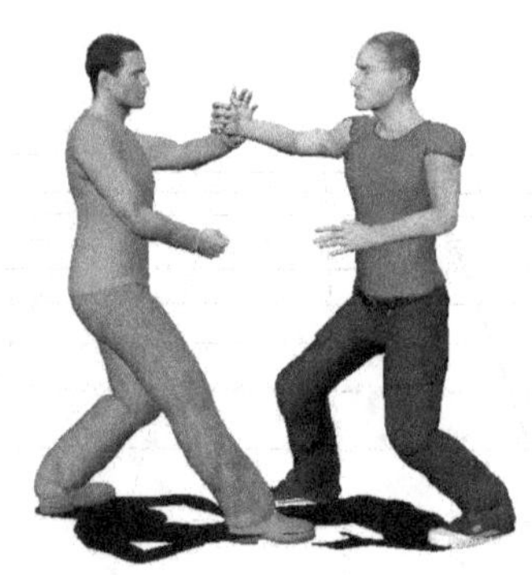

If you leave the Lop Sau sequence you will create an opening for the attacker to exploit.

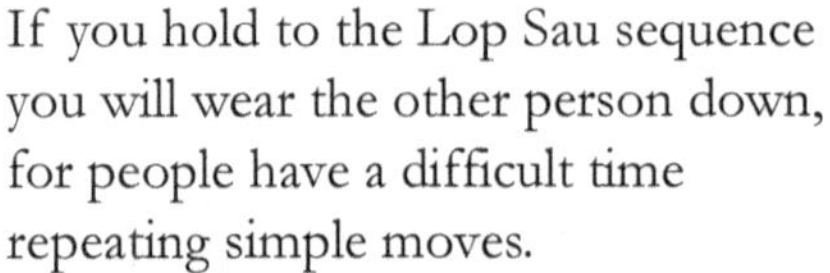

Chapter Twenty-Seven

Lop Sau Grab Arts

The following techniques are done as part of the Lop Sau drill.

They are grab art extensions of the six techniques.

The student should be able to respond with the basic responses

to the six attacks before you teach him these.

You need not wait for him to master attacking.

that will come with time.

While I have a fair grasp on grappling techniques, locks, takedowns, and so on, I never spent much time on those styles.

It is a common saying that all fights end up on the ground, and that is a completely false premise. That is a saying promoted by those who study arts like wrestling and ju jitsu.

But the fact is that fights only go to the ground if you are fighting somebody who specializes in the ground fighting. It fights don't always go to the ground if a person has spent a bit of time studying how not to go to the ground.

Most important, if you allow a fight to go to the ground you are then immobile, a sitting duck for an opponent's friends.

I hope it is obvious that these few techniques can lead to hundreds, if not thousands, of locks, combinations, variations, deviations, and so on.

Elbow Roll/Arm Bar

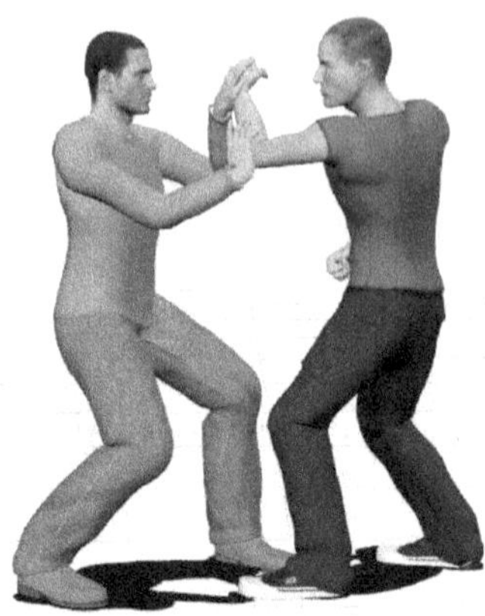

This is the first lop sau grab art I teach. It is applied when the attacker begins rolling his backfist into you.

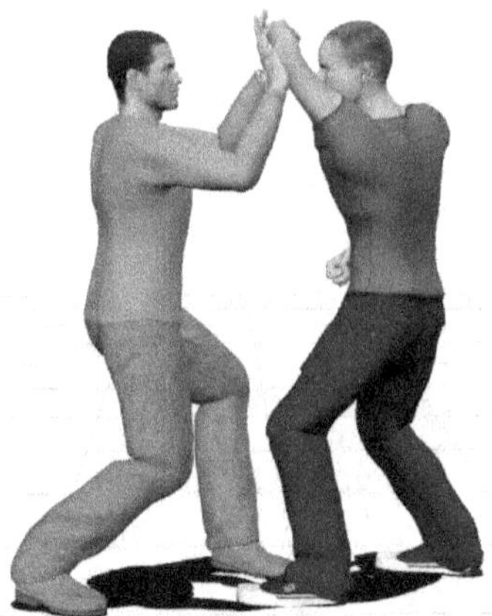

Begin moving forward, catching his wrist with your left hand and pushing up on his elbow with your righthand. This is the beginning of an elbow roll.

If the attacker tries to wiggle out it is very easy to morph into an arm bar.

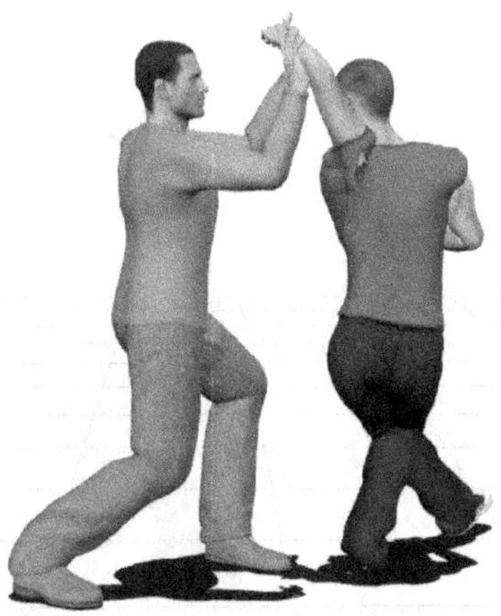

Continue pushing up on his arm…TAKING A STEP FORWARD AS YOU DO SO!

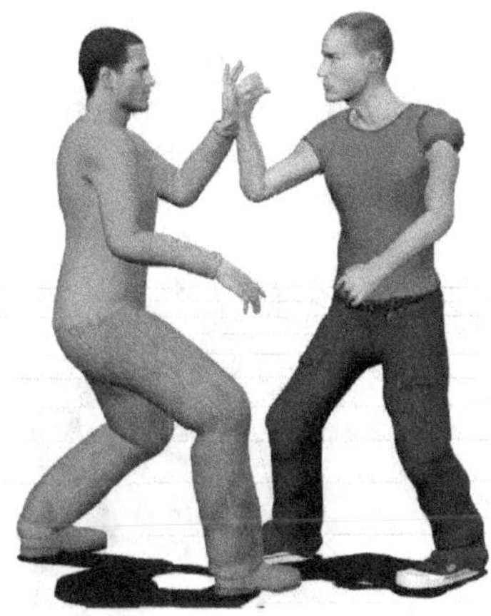

The defender must take a cross step with his right leg, the pivot all the way around to execute a rolling backfist with the other hand, with the stances reverse.

You will find that the attacker sometimes blocks with the wrong hand, which necessitates a second forward push and arm bar.

Arm Wrapping

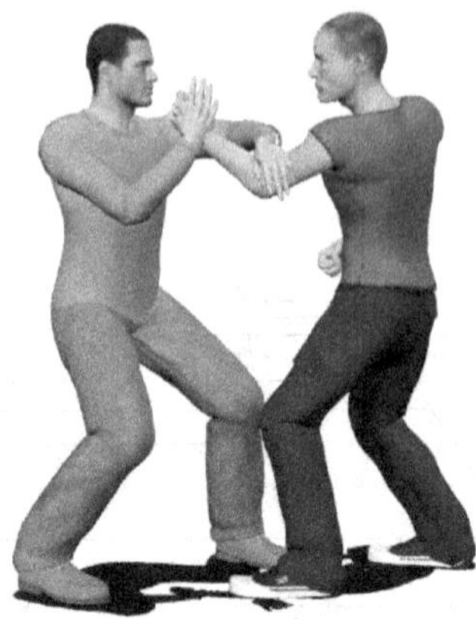

Arm wrapping can be done on the first technique.

When the attacker extends the backfist (jab) to the head put your rear hand up to block, but shoot your front hand over the attacker's elbow crotch and point downward.

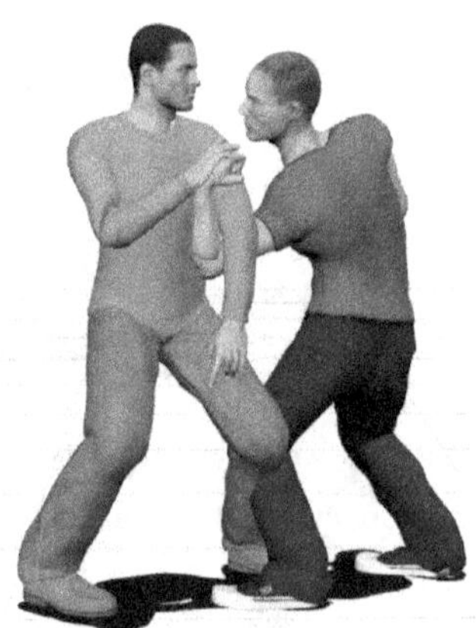

This inverts the attacker's front elbow for a takedown.

Remember to point your finger. This is not a muscle technique, but a quick and relaxed technique.

Please note that the rear hand executes an outward wrist twist to the opponent's front hand.

Vertical Arm Pin

This move works off the first technique.

When the attacker rolls into a backfist, pull it, or do a slap grab to it.

Grabbing the attacker's front wrist execute a slap to the face. Or chop to the neck or backfist to the face, or even a poke to the eyes.

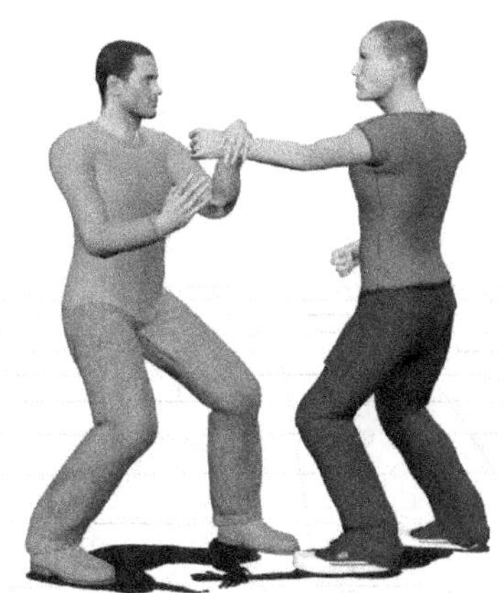

You should be moving forward on the slap to increase the body weight behind your strike.

Keep moving forward as you push the attacker's arm up and around, and his head down.

You will find he will collapse into a pin wheere you hold his arm vertical.

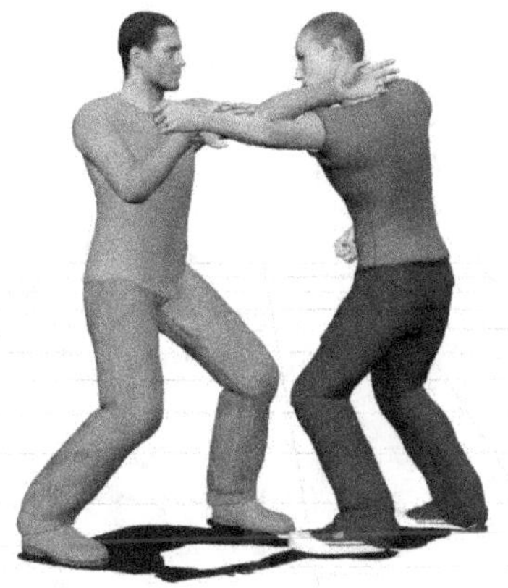

Look for an outward wrist twist to his hand.

DO NOT push his arm straight up.

DO NOT push his arm straight around.

You MUST push his arm in a spiral that is 45 degrees until it is vertical to the ground.

It is possible to do an elbow spike to the head to make the technique work.

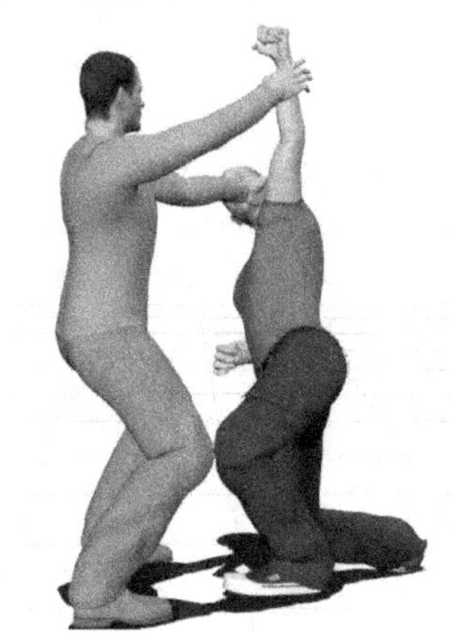

Cross Down

Cross down occurs for a punch to the belly (or a knife), such as in lop sau techniques three and four.

When the partner counters with a body strike simple cross the hands and jam downwards, placing the right arm behind the elbow (able to pull up on the bones) and the left hand down on the wrist.

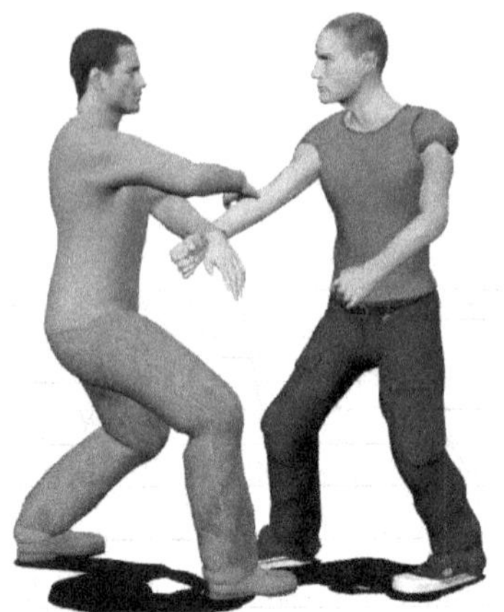

Pull up on the elbow and push down and around on the wrist.

Snake the left arm over the crotch of the elbow and point towards the ground.

At first this technique will be difficult, as the student will apply the cross down technique with force.

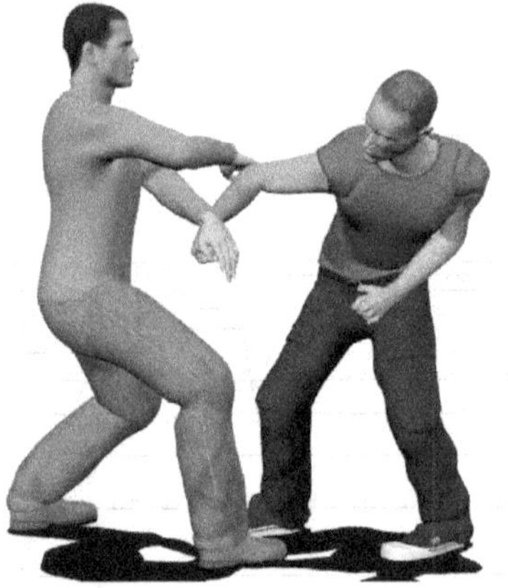

As soon as he learns that he is not stopping, but catching and guiding, then it will be easy.

One thing you should know is that if the partner resists any grab art you may 'soften him uop' with an elbow to the head, a slap to the face, or any other 'shock and lock' move.

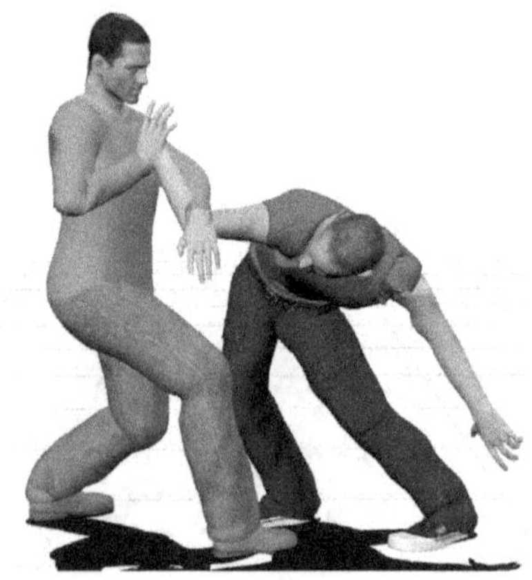

Stripping Grabs

I should tell you the defense for when somebody does a grab art to you.

Strip them.

This means not becoming rigid and resisting, but becoming snakelike, and using your other arm to simply push their grab off.

In the figure to the right the man on the left is pushing an armbar.

The man on the right shifts back and simply pushes up on one or both of the attacker's hands.

To strip simply push or pulled the wrist, or body part doing to pushing, pulling or grabbing.

This comes from the five army theory in Matrix Tai Chi Chuan.

Give way and manipulate the attacker past, or into a disadvantageous position.

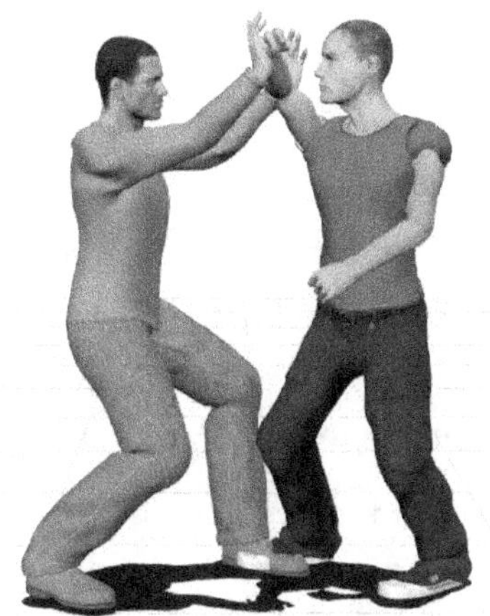

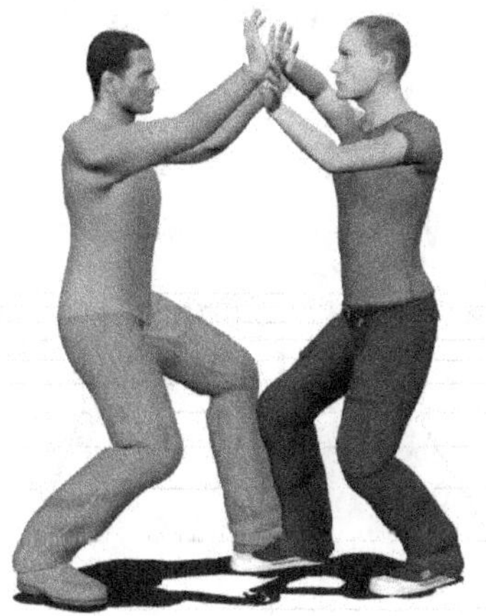

Conclusion

These days the classic arts often get a bad rap.

Bully boys claim it doesn't work in the ring, and they laugh at our techniques.

Often, they are right.

With Matrixing that changes. With matrixing one has the tools to make an art that works

There are no poser techniques, no less than useful techniques, no unrealistic drills and methods.

In this book, Advanced Nine Square diagram Kung Fu,' matrixing has taken the art to a high level.

This art *really* works…but only if you make it work.

Practice, every day. Do your form with closed eyes and open your eyes to a new world. Expand your senses and build your energy.

Find training partners and go over the techniques endlessly.

Most of all, find partners and do Lop Sau, figure out how to evolve into Push Hands, and apply it all to freestyle.

Do not feel you have to jump in a ring and get your face bashed in to learn something.

This art, my instructions followed to the letter, leads to enlightenment.

Which would you rather have? A world that solves problems by brute force? War and physical battles? With the resultant hospitals and smashing of dreams and abilities?

Or higher abilities, and the will to solve problems through reason and imagination?

Have a great work out!

Al Case

Al Case is a ninth degree black belt.

He has written hundreds of books and instruction manuals

Here are a few of those books.

CHIANG NAN

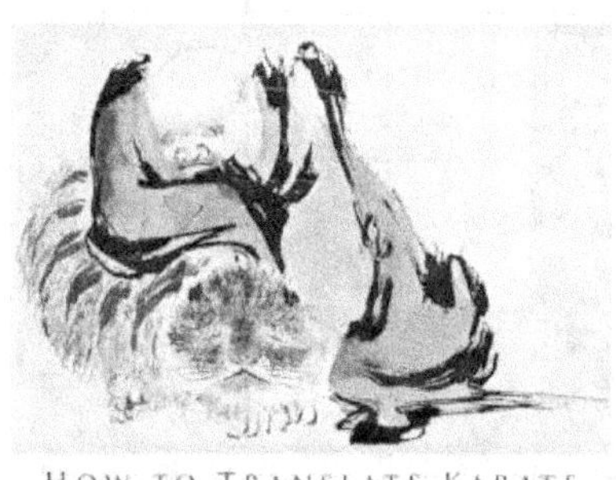

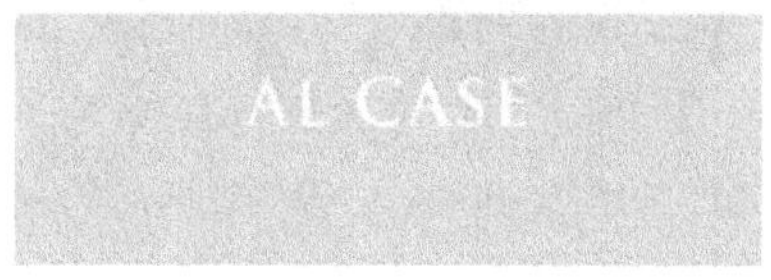

Do Karate Chiang Nan style and you will gain an insight to Karate that has never been available before.

You will learn how to flow techniques, how to gain a type of tai chi energy which I usually refer to as 'suspended energy.

But no matter what I call it, it is a massive boost in chi power, which will improve your body, make it more flexible, stronger, rehabilitate injuries, and definitely give you the long life you deserve.

Chiang Nan

How to translate Karate into Tai Chi Chuan

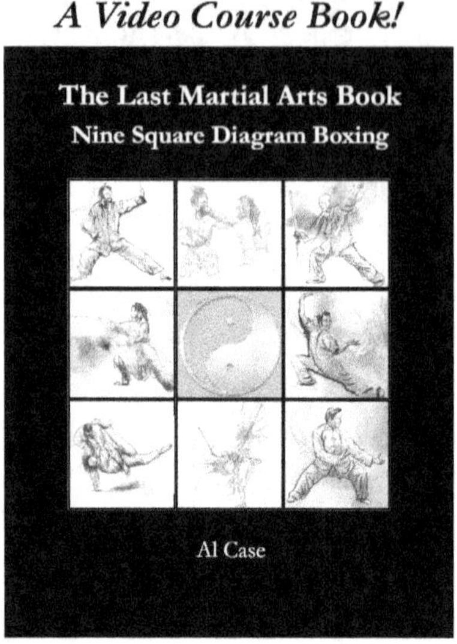

A true tour de force, this book takes its place among the classics of the martial arts!

Includes over 5 hours of videos. All forms, techniques, everything demonstrated on video!

Blends the workability of street wise western Martial Arts with the esoteric meditative aspects of Eastern Martial Arts.

Nine Square Diagram Boxing consists of nine 'techniques,' or forms, which take into account every potential of attack and defense.

The workability of hard core Karate and a heightened 'zen' frame of mind.

The forms are modular, as in Pa Kua Chang. They can be done individually, and yet linked together for an infinite number of possible applications.

Everything is tied together with tight, scientific logic. These are simple forms that breed simple techniques that work in the ring, on the street, or just for your peace of mind.

This is a completely new system, immaculately put together. No missing pieces, no faulty logic, a real work of art.

'The Last Martial Arts Book' is, without a doubt, the BEST Martial Arts Book ever written.

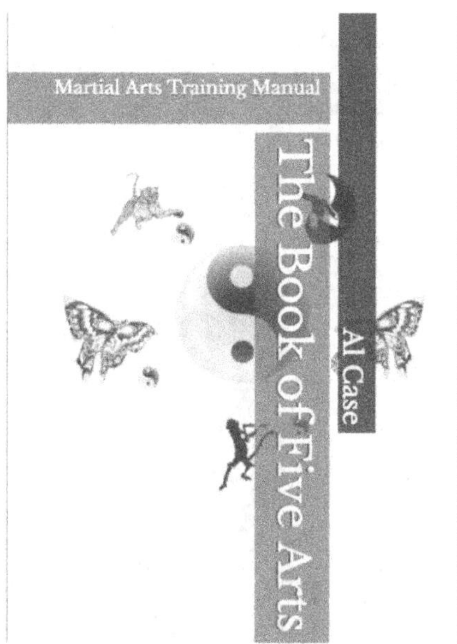

From Al Case, inventor of Matrixing Martial Arts Technology, comes the ultimate Martial Arts book: 'The Book of Five Arts.'

Five martial arts, including forms, two man forms, matrixing charts, showing how the martial arts evolve from had to soft.

In The Book of Five Arts Al has described five arts, enabling the reader to actually go through the martial arts and see the whole picture. This will enable them not to just read about a strategy and wonder how it works, but experience the strategy and KNOW how it works.

There are matrixing charts and procedures throughout the book. These charts take out all the blank spots, enabling the reader to see how to make a martial art perfect.

The reader will be able to use this data to fix his own martial art.

Most important, the reader will finally see the complete procedure for making the martial arts into one art, how they fit together and why.

The book is 164 pages with over 300 illustrations.

Arts include:Matrix Karate/Shaolin Butterfly/Butterfly Pa Kua Chang/ Matrix Tai Chi Chuan/Monkey Boxing

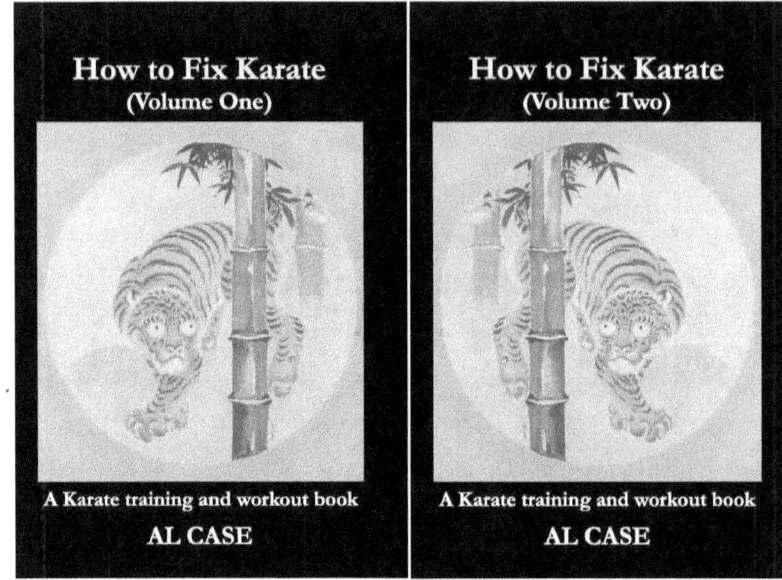

HOW TO FIX KARATE ~ (Two Volumes)

INCLUDE LINKS TO MANY HOURS OF VIDEOS!

Karate has taken a bad rap in recent years. Consider the list of complaints.

It doesn't work in street
It's for children
It's for tournaments
It's too political
The forms don't have anything to do with fighting
The techniques don't have anything to do with fighting
It's too commercial

And the list goes on...

But at one time Karate was the baddest art in the world! Imperial bodyguards from three different countries used it. People could break coconuts with a punch and bricks with a chop. There are even stories of Karate practitioners disarming and defeating armed samurai!

So what happened?
We could point the finger here, commercialism, tournaments, racism, incompetent instructors, politics…but that doesn't really do any good.

Instead, what if we actually fixed karate?

What if, instead of buying into a less than adequate martial art we dissected karate and isolated the working principles?

What if, instead of just doing what we are taught, we start thinking about it, questioning the art.

What if we take apart each and every form, what if we toss out the crap techniques and the poser and dancers and start working on only the techniques that work?

The result would be a karate that worked. A karate where freestyle and forms were not different. A karate with the guts that made it the most formidable martial art in the world!

In the two volumes of 'How to Fix Karate' the author does exactly that. He takes apart the most practice forms of karate and restructures them and… fixes them.

Using physics he analyzes the body and the motions.

Using history and matrixing logic he gets rid of techniques that were created for different weapons, different times and weird reasons.

Forms are restructured. Missing pieces are filled in. BS is tossed out. Mysticism goes on a lo-o-ong vacation.

Techniques are adjusted so they work. Attackers no longer have to wait for the student to 'catch up.' There is no more dancing.

Everything becomes simple and logical.

The truth is this: the mind likes what is simple and logical, and it absorbs such information quickly and easily. Karate, done this way takes a short time to learn, and is intuitive in action. It really starts to work.

Two volumes (must be bought separately)

Over 400 pages
Over 50,000 words
nearly 400 images
over 50 form applications ~ every single move from the forms!
A section on Matrixing that will expand understanding of the forms and techniques!

There are links to videos at the beginning of some chapters, so make sure you retain your receipt in the event that links change.

Has complete data for continuing Karate far beyond Black Belt, and includes A COMPLETE VIDEO COURSE ON FIGHTING.

You can find Al Case Martial Arts books and videos on the net.

Go to MonsterMartialArts.com